CWON®

Exam Practice Questions

Mometrix
TEST PREPARATION

Dear Future Exam Success Story

First of all, **THANK YOU** for purchasing Mometrix study materials!

Second, congratulations! You are one of the few determined test-takers who are committed to doing whatever it takes to excel on your exam. **You have come to the right place.** We developed these practice tests with one goal in mind: to deliver you the best possible approximation of the questions you will see on test day.

Standardized testing is one of the biggest obstacles on your road to success, which only increases the importance of doing well in the high-pressure, high-stakes environment of test day. Your results on this test could have a significant impact on your future, and these practice tests will give you the repetitions you need to build your familiarity and confidence with the test content and format to help you achieve your full potential on test day.

Your success is our success

We would love to hear from you! If you would like to share the story of your exam success or if you have any questions or comments in regard to our products, please contact us at **800-673-8175** or **support@mometrix.com**.

Thanks again for your business and we wish you continued success!

Sincerely,
The Mometrix Test Preparation Team

Written and edited by the Mometrix Exam Secrets Test Prep Team
Printed in the United States of America

TABLE OF CONTENTS

Practice Test #1

Wound Care Practice Questions

1. A solid skin barrier wafer with a pouch is applied to a copiously draining wound, but the skin beneath the wafer has become denuded. The BEST initial solution is to

a. apply a skin barrier powder to the denuded skin under the wafer.
b. discontinue use of the pouch and apply topical dressing.
c. apply a moisture barrier paste under the wafer.
d. apply a moisture barrier ointment to the skin and absorbent dressings.

2. Which of the following biological skin substitutes would be appropriate for repair post-Mohs procedure for a large facial squamous cell carcinoma?

a. Apligraf
b. TransCyte
c. Integra
d. Dermagraft

3. During the phases of healing, which cell is responsible for beginning angiogenesis?

a. neutrophil
b. fibroblast
c. macrophage
d. myofibroblast

4. Which wound dressing type is most likely to result in pain during dressing change?

a. gauze
b. hydrocolloid
c. hydrogel
d. alginates

5. A basic principle of wound care with occlusive dressings is to keep the wound

a. cool and dry
b. warm and dry
c. warm and moist
d. cool and moist

6. The *BEST* candidate for hyperbaric oxygen therapy is a patient with

a. chronic venous ulcers, refractory to standard treatment.
b. chronic diabetic ulcers (Wagner III classification), refractory to standard treatment.
c. newly diagnosed osteomyelitis, recently started on standard treatment.
d. acute wound from trauma to lower leg.

7. Which of the following is the *BEST* debridement choice for an infected diabetic ulcer with hard gray callus formation at wound edges?

a. sharp debridement with saucerization or callus removal
b. autolytic debridement with hydrogels or hydrocolloids
c. autolytic debridement with transparent film dressing
d. enzymatic debridement

8. When using the pinch test as an initial assessment of skin turgor and dehydration, which site provides the most accurate results?

a. skin on top of hand or palm
b. skin on forehead or sternum
c. skin on abdomen
d. skin on forearm or upper arm

9. According to the Modified Wagner Foot Ulcer Classification System, a full-thickness ulcer that extends to the tendon or joint but without abscess or osteomyelitis is classified as

a. grade 1.
b. grade 2.
c. grade 3.
d. grade 4.

10. When using transparent film dressing for autolytic debridement, how often should dressing changes be scheduled?

a. 8 to 10 days
b. 5 to 7 days
c. 3 to 5 days
d. 1 to 2 days

11. A chronic ulcer resulting from peripheral vascular insufficiency may remain in which phase of healing for prolonged periods?

a. hemostasis
b. inflammation
c. proliferation
d. remodeling

12. Hypertrophic scars are *MOST* likely to occur

a. over joints.
b. in dark-skinned patients.
c. on the deltoids and earlobes.
d. on the upper back and chest.

13. When developing a plan of care for a patient who must learn wound management, which of the following would be an appropriate listing of a behavioral outcome?

a. understands the need to do daily dressing change
b. accepts mobility limitations
c. feels that he can manage wound care independently within a few days
d. able to demonstrate dressing change in 3 days

14. A patient has marked bilateral non-pitting edema of both lower legs and feet, including toes, and has thickening of the skin but no pigmentation. This edema can *MOST* likely be characterized as

a. orthostatic edema.
b. lymphedema.
c. lipedema.
d. chronic venous insufficiency.

15. The most common cause of venous outflow obstruction and venous ulceration is

a. deep vein thrombosis.
b. trauma.
c. congestive heart failure.
d. obesity.

16. When applying an Unna boot for a nonhealing venous stasis ulcer, to what tension should the outer self-adhering elastic bandage (Coban) be stretched?

a. 100%
b. 50%
c. 25%
d. 10%

17. Which is the best choice for a support surface for a patient with large stage III and stage IV pressure injuries on multiple turning sites?

a. alternating air mattress
b. static flotation (air)
c. foam
d. low-air-loss therapy device

18. A large open wound on the patient's leg is contaminated with dirt, gravel, and other debris. The *BEST* approach to cleansing is

a. pulsatile lavage only.
b. sharp debridement and pulsatile lavage.
c. hand debridement, large volume irrigation, and pulsatile lavage.
d. large volume irrigation and hand debridement.

19. The presence of necrotic tissue and debris that prevent epithelization from occurring is

a. bioburden.
b. contamination.
c. colonization.
d. critical colonization.

20. Which of the following is the correct documentation of undermining?

a. "Extends 1.8 cm width about one-quarter of wound perimeter."
b. "Extends ¾ inch width by the right lower quadrant of the wound."
c. "Extends 1.8 cm width from 1 o'clock to 4 o'clock."
d. "Extends ¾ inch width from 1 o'clock to 4 o'clock."

21. People with a fluidized air/high-air-loss support surface must be carefully monitored for

a. bottoming.
b. dehydration.
c. fungal infection.
d. tissue maceration.

22. A wound is covered with dry black eschar and is to be debrided with an enzyme. The *FIRST* step is to

a. cover the wound with a layer of enzyme.
b. thoroughly dry the wound.
c. crosshatch through the outer layers of the eschar.
d. do a sharp debridement of the outer layers of the eschar.

23. Which of the following topical antibiotics is the *BEST* choice for a wound that may be infected with bacteria and fungi?

a. cadexomer iodine
b. metronidazole
c. mupirocin
d. silver sulfadiazine 7%

24. Painless open ulcers on the pressure points on the bottom of the foot surrounded by calloused skin usually indicate

a. arterial insufficiency.
b. neuropathy.
c. chronic venous insufficiency.
d. malignancy.

25. Which functional assessment tool measures the 8 activities necessary for an adult to function independently?

a. Barthel Index of Activities of Daily Living
b. Instrumental Activities of Daily Living (IADL)
c. Index of Independence in Activities of Daily Living (Katz Index)
d. Palliative Performance Scale

26. Which therapy is the *MOST* essential for a patient living alone with diabetic peripheral neuropathy and reduced sensation in the hands and feet, resulting in repeated injuries?

a. occupational therapy
b. physical therapy
c. nutritional therapy
d. cognitive-behavioral therapy

27. The nurse places her hand under a 1.5-inch foam overlay and finds that the overlay has compressed to 0.75 inches, indicating

a. bottoming out.
b. adequate support.
c. excess wear.
d. moisture retention.

28. Which dietary modification is *MOST* important to promote healing for a 50-year-old overweight man who has a third-degree burn on his left arm that has had wound debridement and skin grafting?

a. decreased fats
b. increased protein
c. increased carbohydrate
d. decreased calories

29. Using the Payne-Martin classification system for skin tear, how would a skin tear be classified that is characterized by partial-thickness injury with 20% of epidermal flap missing?

a. Category I—Linear type
b. Category I—Flap type
c. Category II—Scant tissue loss type
d. Category III—Complete loss of tissue

30. Which type of healing would be used for a wound with full-thickness skin loss with wound margins that cannot be approximated and with nonviable wound edges?

a. superficial wound healing
b. primary intention
c. delayed primary intention
d. secondary intention

31. If a patient's prealbumin level was 16 mg/dL on admission but current testing shows a level of 10 mg/dL, what does this suggest?

a. indication of acute inadequate protein intake
b. indication of chronic inadequate protein intake
c. level within normal limits
d. indication of infectious process

32. A patient who is receiving oral iron because of an iron deficiency should also be prescribed

a. vitamin A.
b. vitamin C.
c. folate.
d. vitamin D.

33. What is the National Pressure Injury Advisory Panel (NPIAP) staging of a pressure injury that is 6 cm in circumference at the surface, but the base is covered with slough and hard, dry brown-black eschar?

a. Stage II
b. Stage III
c. Stage IV
d. Unstageable

34. When irrigating a wound, what wound irrigation pressure is needed to effectively cleanse the wound while avoiding trauma?

a. < 4 psi
b. 20 to 30 psi
c. 10 to 15 psi
d. > 15 psi

35. Which type of precautions require that the nurse assistant wear a mask while caring for the patient, that the patient be separated from other patients by at least 3 feet with a curtain separating them, and that a patient mask is used during transport?

a. standard
b. contact
c. airborne
d. droplet

36. A patient with Charcot arthropathy who has had 2 weeks of compression to reduce edema and inflammation will probably next need

a. total contact cast.
b. half shoe.
c. removable cast walker.
d. foam dressings for cushioning.

37. Which of the following is the most effective to prevent pressure injuries on the heels?

a. foam heel pads
b. heel dressings
c. heel elevation device
d. sheepskin heel pads

38. Which is the best way to move a patient up in bed in order to prevent shear?

a. place hands under patient's axillary region and pull toward the head of the bed
b. ask patient to use trapeze to pull himself/herself up in bed
c. use a lift/turning sheet to move patient toward the head of the bed
d. lower the head of the bed and elevate the knees and ask patient to slide upward

39. The initial treatment to relieve the itching and prevent excoriation resulting from venous dermatitis is

a. topical antihistamine.
b. compression therapy.
c. topical steroids.
d. topical antibiotics.

40. Which of the following topical treatments is usually the *BEST* choice to reduce infection and odor in a fungating necrotic neoplastic lesion?

a. Dakin's solution
b. yogurt
c. hydrogen peroxide
d. metronidazole

41. The primary problem with using the troughing technique to manage a posterior small bowel fistula in an open abdominal wound is

a. adherence.
b. wound contamination.
c. skin excoriation.
d. fungal infection.

42. When assessing a surgical wound on postoperative day 9, the nurse finds no evidence of a healing ridge. What is the primary implication?

a. wound is healing slowly
b. wound is infected
c. wound is at risk of dehiscence or infection
d. wound is well healed.

43. What is the primary purpose for applying elbow pads to a patient who exhibits repetitive movement of the arms and legs?

a. prevent pressure injuries
b. promote comfort
c. reduce friction
d. reduce shear

44. When cleansing a wound in a shower, how far away from the wound should the showerhead be?

a. 6 inches
b. 2 inches
c. 24 inches
d. 12 inches

45. With static compression therapy, how much pressure should high-level compression dressings exert at the ankle?

a. 30 to 40 mm Hg
b. ≤ 50 mm Hg
c. 10 to 20 mm Hg
d. < 23 mm Hg

46. With Ayello's ASSESSMENTS tool for evaluation of wounds, the "M" refers to

a. marginal edges.
b. medications.
c. management.
d. maceration.

47. When obtaining a wound culture for anaerobic organisms, what should the nurse do immediately after aspirating exudate from deep within the wound?

a. squirt the exudate directly into a culture tube
b. apply a needle to the syringe and expel all air, then inject the exudate into a culture tube
c. apply a needle to the syringe and inject the exudate into a culture tube
d. inject the exudate onto a sterile swab and insert that into a culture tube

48. Which of the following findings on assessment is a risk factor for malnutrition and impaired healing?

a. weight 95% of ideal body weight for age
b. wears dentures
c. drinks 1 to 2 glasses of wine daily
d. body mass index (BMI) of < 18.5

49. Which of the following is an extrinsic factor that may affect wound healing?

a. wound bioburden
b. age
c. nutrition
d. immunosuppression

50. Which of the following wound types would be the *BEST* candidate for negative pressure wound therapy (NPWT)?

a. second-degree burns on arm
b. open wound on leg with osteomyelitis
c. stage III pressure injury with moderate amount exudate
d. abdominal wound dehiscence with organs exposed

51. What is the primary advantage of the clock method of measuring a wound as opposed to the greatest length by greatest width (GLBGW) method?

a. GLBGW underestimates wound size and clock method does not
b. clock method is the most commonly used
c. clock method requires less precision
d. clock method tracks the same site

52. When testing a diabetic patient's vibratory perception threshold (VPT) with a tuning fork, the nurse should first conduct a preliminary test on the patient's

a. lower leg.
b. forehead.
c. forearm.
d. sternum.

53. The primary risk factor for development of pressure injuries is

a. sensory loss.
b. inactivity.
c. immobility.
d. cognitive impairment.

54. When assessing a wound, what is the best way to differentiate between granulation tissue and muscle tissue?

a. observe for color
b. measure temperature difference
c. observe for location in wound
d. palpate and gently pinch tissue

55. Which is the best choice for mechanical debridement of a large infected pressure injury on the right hip with undermining and tunneling in a febrile patient who is undergoing cardiac monitoring?

a. pulsatile lavage with suction
b. whirlpool
c. wet to dry dressing
d. flush with 35 mL syringe with size 19 needle

56. The 5 Ps of neurovascular assessment are

a. pain, pulselessness, position, paresthesia, paraplegia
b. pain, pallor, pulselessness, paresthesia, paraplegia
c. pain, perception, pulselessness, position, paresthesia
d. pain, pulselessness, perception, pallor, paraplegia

57. When doing a continuous wave Doppler probe assessment of peripheral pulses, the normal phasic flow pattern is

a. quadriphasic.
b. triphasic.
c. biphasic.
d. monophasic.

58. What is the *BEST* debridement choice for a venous ulcer with hard brown adherent eschar covering 60% of the wound?

a. autolytic with hydrogels
b. autolytic with transparent film dressing
c. sharp
d. enzymatic

59. What does it mean if the wound surface appears gelatinous 1 week after Apligraf has been applied to a diabetic ulcer?

a. infection
b. rejection
c. allergic response
d. normal response

60. According to Krasner's Chronic Wound Pain Experience (CWPE) model, what intervention would be specifically instituted to relieve cyclic acute wound pain?

a. transcutaneous nerve stimulation
b. tricyclic antidepressants
c. soaking dressing to loosen prior to removal
d. application of heat

61. Which pressure measurement is indicative of limb ischemia?

a. ankle pressure < 60 mm Hg
b. ankle pressure < 40 mm Hg
c. toe pressure < 60 mm Hg
d. toe pressure < 40 mm Hg

62. High-compression stockings (50 to 60 mm Hg), class IV, are recommended for

a. edema associated with venous insufficiency.
b. edema associated with lymphedema.
c. dependent edema.
d. edema with ulceration.

63. What is the *BEST* treatment for a patient with peripheral edema whose lower legs are dry, scaly, and pruritic, resulting in slight excoriation from scratching?

a. warm mineral oil
b. corticosteroid ointment
c. domeboro soaks
d. Neosporin

64. What is the primary purpose of applying foam dressing over amorphous hydrogels or alginates for a large pressure injury?

a. provide protection
b. provide cushioning
c. prevent adherence to the wound
d. remove excess exudate and promote autolysis

65. Which of the following treatments may be used to reduce hypergranulation in a wound?

a. povidone iodine
b. hyaluronic acid (Hyalofill)
c. hypertonic sodium chloride
d. silver sulfadiazine

66. Which is the *BEST* dressing to apply to protect reddened but intact skin in order to prevent skin breakdown?

a. foam dressings
b. hydrocolloids or film dressings
c. sheet hydrogel
d. silver dressings

67. When using a lidocaine soak to prevent pain during debridement of an ulcer, how long should the soak be in contact with the wound before beginning debridement?

a. 3 to 5 minutes
b. 10 to 15 minutes
c. 20 minutes
d. 30 minutes

68. Pressure dressings to prevent scarring are usually indicated when a wound takes longer than

a. > 7 days to heal.
b. > 14 days to heal.
c. > 21 days to heal.
d. > 28 days to heal.

69. When exercising and stretching a scar, maximal stretch is usually indicated by

a. onset of pain.
b. reddening of scar.
c. blanching of scar.
d. increase in pain.

70. In the acute surgical wound, signs of inflammation are normal for the first

a. 24 hours.
b. 2 days.
c. 3 days.
d. 4 days.

71. A patient with a Braden score of 13 has what chance of developing a pressure injury?

a. no risk (normal finding)
b. slight risk (50% to 60%)
c. moderate risk (65% to 90%)
d. high risk (90% to 100%)

72. How many pillows should be placed for pillow bridging to position patients with minimal compression of tissue?

a. 2
b. 3
c. 4
d. 5

73. When assessing venous refill time, venous occlusion is indicated with times of

a. > 3 seconds
b. > 10 seconds
c. > 20 seconds
d. > 30 seconds

74. What intervention is appropriate for a patient with a diabetic ulcer on the great toe, which is swollen, draining, painful, and has purple discoloration?

a. referral to surgeon
b. sharp debridement
c. autolytic debridement
d. enzymatic debridement

75. The Harris mat is used for

a. strengthening exercises.
b. temperature testing to evaluate Charcot's arthropathy.
c. pressure testing for plantar offloading.
d. foot measurements to evaluate swelling.

76. Patients with peripheral neuropathy should have professional skin and nail care of the foot

a. every 2 weeks.
b. weekly.
c. every 2 months.
d. monthly.

77. What is the *BEST* emollient to apply to protect the feet of patients with peripheral neuropathy?

a. petrolatum jelly
b. zinc oxide
c. Vicks VapoRub
d. lotion

78. What is the most likely cause of itching, erythema, scales, and fissures between the toes and on the planter foot surface of a patient who has been taking a broad-spectrum antibiotic for an infected venous ulcer?

a. allergic dermatitis
b. bacterial infection
c. tinea pedis
d. circulatory impairment

79. Which patient is an appropriate candidate for electrical stimulation (ES) therapy?

a. patient with neoplastic wound
b. patient with osteomyelitis
c. 2-year-old patient with burns
d. patient with chronic neuropathic ulcer

80. What transcutaneous oxygen pressure ($tcPO_2$) level indicates that a wound will probably not heal?

a. < 20 mm Hg
b. < 25 mm Hg
c. < 30 mm Hg
d. < 35 mm Hg

Wound Care Answers and Explanations

1. A: A skin barrier powder is used as an initial barrier on denuded skin to provide an adherent base for ointments, pastes, or solid skin adhesive barriers. The powder is sprinkled over the denuded area and excess removed before application of a second barrier. The powder should be applied thinly because excess will impair adhesion of other barrier products, and it should not be used on intact skin because it will not properly adhere. Skin barrier powders contain powder pectin, karaya, gelatin, carboxymethyl cellulose, or combinations. Skin barrier powders are frequently used with ostomy products when the skin has become weepy.

2. C: Integra, with a protective silicone outer layer over a collagen and chondroitin-6-sulfate layer, is FDA approved for a wide variety of uses, including full-thickness or partial-thickness burns, pressure injuries, venous ulcers, diabetic ulcers, and surgical wounds, such as post-Mohs procedure. It is also used to resurface scars and keloids and for contracture release. Integra is usually meshed (1:1 ratio) to allow for drainage and penetration of antimicrobials. After application, Integra is secured with compression dressing or negative pressure.

3. B: During the inflammation phase, macrophages release growth factors, which attract fibroblasts to the wound. Fibroblasts are responsible for beginning angiogenesis and are critically important during the proliferation phase of healing, which usually begins at about day 3 after trauma. In addition to angiogenesis, fibroblasts initiate formation of collagen (type III) and initiate epithelialization, which begins from the basement membrane of the skin or from the wound edges if the basement membrane is compromised.

4. A: Gauze dressings cause the most pain during dressing changes because they tend to adhere to the wound when dry. Even though wet-to-dry gauze dressings are frequently prescribed, they may result in trauma to the wound, damaging granulating tissue, and should be avoided in favor of dressing types that maintain a moist environment. The primary considerations when choosing a dressing type should be those that cause the least wound trauma and the least pain while promoting healing.

5. C: Occlusive dressings should keep the wound warm and moist. Reasons include:

- Reduction in dehydration allows cells such as neutrophils and fibroblasts to carry out their functions in wound repair. This also results in less cell death.
- Angiogenesis requires a moist environment and low oxygen tension.
- Autolytic debridement with proteolytic enzymes is enhanced.
- Re-epithelization of tissue occurs because the epidermal cells are able to spread across the surface of the wound.
- Reduction in microorganisms because the seal provided by occlusive dressings decreases infection.
- Pain reduction results from the protection of nerve endings and the need for fewer dressing changes.

6. B: The best candidate for hyperbaric oxygen therapy is the patient with chronic diabetic ulcers (Wagner classification III or higher), refractory to standard treatment. During treatment, patients breathe 100% oxygen in a pressurized environment. Hyperbaric oxygen therapy increases available oxygen to tissues by 10 to 20 times. Blood that is saturated increases perfusion of the tissues. Hyperbaric oxygen therapy is indicated for peripheral arterial insufficiency, compromised skin from grafts, and diabetic ulcers (usually Wagner III or higher). In 2003, Medicare approved payment for hyperbaric oxygen therapy to treat diabetic ulcers.

7. A: Sharp debridement with saucerization (tissue excavated to form a shallow depression to facilitate drainage) is the best choice for an infected diabetic ulcer with callus formation, although repeat saucerization may be required with each dressing change. All of the callus and necrotic tissue should be removed and the wound flushed with sterile saline. In some cases, autolytic debridement with hydrocolloids or hydrogels may be used first to help soften the callus prior to its removal.

8. B: The pinch test is not very reliable for assessing dehydration, especially if done over areas with much subcutaneous tissue, so the best sites are on the forehead or over the sternum. Indications of dehydration include cracked lips, dry mucous membranes, tachycardia, altered sensations, hypotension, and weight loss. If dehydration is suspected, then it should be confirmed with diagnostic testing, such as serum osmolality, serum sodium, BUN, BUN/creatinine ratio, urine specific gravity, and albumin.

9. B: A full-thickness ulcer that extends to the tendon or joint but without abscess or osteomyelitis is classified as grade 2. The Modified Wagner Foot Ulcer Classification System separates foot ulcers into 6 grades (grade 0 to grade 5). Classification is based on depth of lesion, presence of osteomyelitis, gangrene, infection, ischemia, and neuropathy, but does not include ulcer size, so this grading system is not used in isolation; however, it is predictive of outcomes, with grades 3 to 4 indicating marked compromise.

10. C: Transparent film should be changed every 3 to 5 days, although the dressing should always be changed if leakage occurs as this can cause tissue maceration. Transparent film is most useful for dry eschar, which should be crosshatched prior to application of the film to facilitate autolysis. The dressing should be at least 2 inches larger than the size of the wound. The wound should be irrigated with NS and a skin sealant applied to surrounding tissue prior to application of the dressing.

11. B: Chronic ulcers with poor perfusion or other complicating factors, such as infection, may remain in the inflammatory phase of healing. If the macrophages that are activated during the inflammation stage are not able to adequately attract fibroblasts, then the angiogenesis, formation of collagen, and epithelization that are necessary for the wound to heal do not take place, so the wound remains stalled for long periods of time unless the complicating factors are aggressively treated and reversed.

12. A: Hypertrophic scars most frequently occur over joints where there is tension on the wound. They remain localized to the area of the original wound and may spontaneously regress. They may result in contracture of the wound. Keloid scars most frequently occur on the upper back and chest as well as the deltoids and earlobes. They extend beyond the original wound and rarely regress. They usually arise after the wound has healed as raised, shiny, rope-like fibrous scars. They do not result in contracture of the wound.

13. D: Behavioral outcomes should always be measureable, such as "able to demonstrate dressing change in 3 days." This outcome covers a specific task and a time frame, making it easy to evaluate. Words such as "understands," "accepts," and "feels," are not measureable. Behavioral outcomes should be described in terms of actions words, such as "demonstrates," "states," "describes," and "lists." Behavioral outcomes should always be those things that can be directly observed and measured to determine if outcomes have been successfully achieved within the allotted time.

14. B: Lymphedema: Hard, nonpitting edema with skin thickening but no pigmentation. Edema usually includes the feet and toes and often occurs bilaterally. Orthostatic edema: Occurs with prolonged sitting and is soft and pitting but without skin thickening or pigmentation. It is always bilateral and includes edema of the foot. Lipedema: Bilateral fatty deposition in legs may mimic edema, but there is no pitting, skin thickening, or pigmentation, and no edema of the foot. Chronic venous insufficiency: Edema is soft and pitting initially but may harden later. Skin thickening may occur around the ankles and pigmentation changes are common. Edema often involves feet and may be bilateral.

15. A: The most common cause of venous outflow obstruction and venous ulceration is deep vein thrombosis. With obstruction, veins distal to the obstructed area become distended, resulting in increased venous hypertension (sustained increased pressure in the legs). As the venous pressure rises, venous stasis occurs, leading to ulceration. Other factors that can also contribute to increased venous hypertension include obesity, CHF, edema, trauma, ascites, and tumors of the legs.

16. B: An Unna boot is used to treat nonhealing stasis ulcers in ambulatory patients. If the ulcer is draining, it should be packed with alginate, and a dressing should be applied to absorb the discharge until the Unna boot is changed. Before applying, the leg and ulcers should be cleaned, and the leg should be patted dry. Most wraps contain a moisture barrier, generally, zinc oxide and glycerin. The wrap must be applied upward from the toes to about 1 inch below the knee. It is then covered with an elastic bandage or self-adhering bandage (such as Coban), stretched to 50% tension.

17. D: The best choice for a patient with large stage III and stage IV pressure injuries on multiple turning sites is a low-air-loss therapy device. Low-air-loss devices may use a bed frame or be placed on top of a standard mattress. Low-air-loss therapy devices have low moisture retention, reduced heat accumulation, and provide relief of pressure in any position, so they are particularly useful for patients with multiple pressure injuries. The devices comprise connected air-filled pillows covered by a low-friction material. The amount of air and pressure in each pillow can be separately calibrated.

18. C: Foreign material should be removed by hand debridement from a large open contaminated wound followed by large-volume irrigation at 5 to 8 lb pressure per square inch (usually using a < 19-gauge needle) and pulsatile lavage in order to reduce the risk of infection. Pulsatile high-pressure lavage is irrigation of an infected or necrotic wound under pressure, using an electrically powered device. Normal saline is commonly used for lavage treatments, with the amount varying according to the size and amount of exudate on the wound. It is recommended that pressure be between 8 to 15 psi.

19. A: Bioburden refers to the presence of necrotic tissue and debris that prevent epithelialization from occurring. Bioburden contributes to the development of infection in the wound. Contamination of a wound means that bacteria are present but are not multiplying. Colonization is common and occurs when bacteria multiply in the wound but do not cause an inflammatory response, damage tissues, or retard healing. Critical colonization occurs when bacteria replicate to a level that causes delay in healing without causing an inflammatory response or an infection with tissue damage.

20. C: Undermining, which is damaged tissue under intact skin, usually occurs around the perimeter of a wound. Undermining is reported in centimeters and in relation to the open wound by reference to a clock face: "extends 1.8 cm width from 1 o'clock to 4 o'clock." If the undermining is open, it can be measured by insertion of a sterile swab. In some cases, tissue may be damaged but remains intact; in that case, undermining is estimated by palpation as undermined tissue may feel spongy.

21. B: The increased airflow with fluidized air/high-air-loss support surfaces can increase evaporative fluid loss, so patients must be adequately hydrated to compensate and avoid dehydration. Intake and output must be carefully monitored, and skin turgor and mucous membranes must be evaluated. Fluidized air/high-air-loss support surfaces have beads with a pH of 10 (alkaline), so they have bacteriocidal properties, decreasing risk of infection. These support surfaces reduce friction, shear, and pressure, as well as moisture, decreasing risk of fungal infection.

22. C: Because enzymes require a moist environment, the first step when treating dry eschar is to crosshatch through the outer layers of the eschar. Chemical debridement with enzymes, such as collagenase and papain/urea, is effective for wounds with necrosis and eschar but may take several days to several weeks to debride a large area of eschar. Various types of dressing can be used with enzymes, but they must be easily removable because enzymes must be applied one to two times daily.

23. A: Cadexomer iodine is effective against a wide range of bacteria (*S. aureus,* MRSA, *Streptococcus,* and *Pseudomonas)*, viruses, and fungi. Metronidazole: Effective against bacterial infections. Mupirocin: Effective against gram-positive organisms (such as *S. aureus* and MRSA*)* and may be used to treat nasal colonization, which increases risk of wound infection. Silver sulfadiazine 7%: Effective against gram-positive organisms, including *S. aureus,* MRSA, *Streptococcus,* and *Pseudomonas.* Topical antibiotics provide effective reduction of surface pathogens but can result in systemic reactions, so patients must be monitored carefully. The same antibiotic should not be used for both systemic and topical treatment because this increases risk of resistance.

24. B: Painless open ulcers on the pressure areas on the bottom of the foot surrounded by calloused skin indicate neuropathic ulcers, such as those commonly found with diabetic polyneuropathy. Because of reduced sensation, patients may develop ulcers from chronic pressure (indicated by the callus formation) without noticing, especially if they do not check their feet or are unable to do so. The nylon monofilament test can be used to assess the patient's degree of protective sensation.

25. B: Instrumental Activities of Daily Living (IADL): An assessment tool to measure 8 activities necessary for an adult to function independently. This tool helps to determine the need for supportive services. Barthel Index of Activities of Daily Living: Assesses the functional ability of older adults in 10 categories. It is used to assess the person's disabilities and need for assistance. Index of Independence in Activities of Daily Living (Katz Index): Evaluates 6 areas to provide an assessment of the person's need for assistance and progression of disease and/or disability. Palliative Performance Scale: Assesses the functional ability of older adults receiving palliative care.

26. A: Occupational therapy assists patients with home safety and self-care issues, such as wearing properly fitted shoes, checking skin, safe walking, cooking modifications, and housecleaning techniques to minimize injury. Injuries are common with peripheral neuropathy because of reduced sensation. Physical therapy may also be helpful to maintain range of motion and increase strength. Nutritional therapy should be part of all diabetic teaching. Cognitive-behavioral therapy works toward solving particular behavioral problems by increasing awareness and developing strategies, but the injuries are related to sensory changes more than behavioral problems.

27. A: Support surface material should provide at least an inch of support under areas to be protected when in use to prevent "bottoming out." When determining the type of overlay, the patient's size and weight must be considered. Generally, all patients at risk should have some type of pressure-reducing overlay on their beds. Viscoelastic foam provides some protection and may protect from shear and friction. Other nondynamic overlays, such as those made with foam chips, tend to deteriorate faster than viscoelastic foam.

28. B: Increased protein is especially important for wound healing. The average healthy person requires about 0.8 g of protein per kilogram every day (40 to 70 g). However, if a person has a wound, then the person must have adequate calories and general nutrition daily as well as added protein and vitamins as well. Protein amounts are increased to 1.25 to 2 g/kg to promote healing. Healing requires extra calories as well, but ensuring a high protein nutritious diet is more important than simply reducing calories or fat or increasing carbohydrates.

29. C: Category II—Scant tissue loss type. Payne-Martin Categories:

Category I: Skin tear without tissue loss:

- Linear: Full-thickness wound in wrinkle or furrow with epidermis and dermis pulled apart (incisional appearance).
- Flap: Partial-thickness wound with a flap that can cover wound with ≤ 1 mm of dermis exposed.

Category II: Skin tear with partial tissue loss.

- Scant tissue loss: Partial-thickness injury and ≤ 25% of epidermal flap lost.
- Moderate-large tissue loss: Partial-thickness injury with > 25% epidermal flap lost.

Category III: Skin tear with complete tissue loss.

- Complete partial-thickness injury with loss of epidermal flap.

30. D: Wounds that involve full-thickness skin loss with margins that cannot be approximated and/or have nonviable wound edges are usually left to heal by secondary intention. In some cases of large wounds, skin grafting may be required. Secondary intention healing is also indicated for grossly contaminated wounds that carry a high risk of infection and necrotic tissue. The wound is covered with a dressing and left to heal through regeneration rather than repair, resulting in scar tissue and contraction.

31. A: Prealbumin is used to assess acute changes in nutritional status, so a decrease from 16 to 10 mg/dL indicates that the patient has had recent acute inadequate protein intake, possibly because of the increased demand for protein and calories to promote healing. Because prealbumin's half-life is only 2 to 3 days, it can change rapidly in response to nutritional changes:

- Normal value: 16-40 mg/dL.
- Mild deficiency: 10-15 mg/dL
- Moderate deficiency: 5-9 mg/dL.
- Severe deficiency: < 5 mg/dL.

This patient's diet should be reevaluated and protein and calories increased to meet the increased needs.

32. B: Patients taking oral iron should also take vitamin C because it increases the iron absorption. Dosage is usually equivalent to or higher than the iron dosage. Vitamin C also promotes the formation of collagen and promotes wound healing, so deficiency can result in impaired healing and increased capillary fragility. Ferrous sulfate is usually used for iron deficiency in adults, with dosage varying according to hemoglobin and other factors. Patients should receive nutritional counseling regarding foods high in iron and vitamin C.

33. D: Because injury to tissues may be more extensive than what is visible with a pressure injury, a pressure injury in which the base cannot be visualized must be staged as "unstageable" with the NPIAP Pressure Injury Staging until the wound can be adequately debrided and the base examined to determine depth. The base may be obscured by slough of various colors (yellow to brown) or eschar (brown or black). To ensure proper treatment, a wound classified as unstageable should be debrided and restaged as soon as possible.

34. C: Wounds should be irrigated with pressures of 10 to 15 psi. An irrigation pressure of < 4 psi does not adequately cleanse a wound, and pressures > 15 psi can result in trauma to the wound, interfering with healing. A mechanical irrigation device is more effective for irrigation than a bulb syringe, which delivers about ≤ 2 psi. A 250 mL squeeze bottle supplies about 4.5 psi, adequate for low-pressure cleaning. A 35 mL syringe with a 19-gauge needle provides about 8 psi.

35. D: Transmission-based precautions include:

Contact	Use personal protective equipment (PPE), including gown and gloves, for all contacts with the patient or patient's immediate environment.
	Maintain patient in private room or > 3 feet away from other patients.
Droplet	Use mask while caring for the patient. Maintain patient in a private room or > 3 feet away from other patients with curtain separating them.
	Use patient mask if transporting patient from one area to another.
Airborne	Place patient in an airborne infection isolation room.
	Use ⍰ N95 respirators (or masks) while caring for patient.

36. A: Charcot arthropathy should be treated with total contact cast for months, with duration depending on the location of the deformity: 12 months for hindfoot, 9 months for midfoot, and 6 months for forefoot. The casts should be changed weekly during the time the volume is changing and then every 2 to 3 weeks. Temperatures should be checked on both sides and should be within 3°F after recalcification. The patient may be allowed gradual weight-bearing after skin has resumed normal temperature.

37. C: The only way to prevent pressure on the heels is to elevate the heel so that it is not in contact with a surface, such as the bed or wheelchair footrest. A special heel elevation device can be utilized, or a pillow may be placed under the legs to elevate the heels. Additionally, a pillow should be placed between the ankles to prevent pressure injuries where the feet contact each other. The patient's position should be changed frequently with full-body turning to 30-degree lateral position, avoiding side-lying.

38. C: Because shear results from a combination of friction and pressure, the only safe way to avoid shear when moving a patient up in bed is to use a lift/turning sheet with two people lifting and moving the patient toward the head of the bed. If possible, the patient can assist by utilizing a trapeze, but the patient should avoid pulling himself/herself toward the head of the bed with the trapeze unless the patient is able to lift completely off the bed with the feet placed flat on the bed to avoid shear on the heels.

39. A: Venous dermatitis appears on the ankles and lower legs and can cause severe itching and pain, and without treatment to control the dermatitis, it may deteriorate, causing ulcers to form, so treatment is needed to alleviate the symptoms. Initial treatment is usually with topical antihistamines. If this does not relieve symptoms, then low-dose topical steroids may be used for short periods only (2 weeks) to reduce inflammation and itching because of the danger of increasing ulceration.

40. D: Metronidazole, in gel or solution, has proven to be an effective topical treatment to control infection and odor in necrotic tumors because it is effective against a wide range of anaerobic bacteria. The solution is used to irrigate the wound, and the gel is applied directly to the tissue. Hydrogen peroxide may irritate the tissue while Dakin's solution has an odor that some patients dislike, although both may reduce tumor odor. Some people have used yogurt and buttermilk topically to reduce odor by reducing wound pH, but there is little research to support their use.

41. B: Troughing is one method of fistula management that is appropriate for fistulas in the posterior aspect of an abdominal wound; however, this technique does not protect the wound from exudate, so the wound can become contaminated. Troughing involves applying skin barrier wafer to the skin surrounding the wound and skin barrier paste to the edges. Then, thin film dressing is applied to the wound down to the fistula opening and an ostomy pouch is cut to fit and applied about the fistula opening. This method allows drainage from the wound and the fistula to mix as they both drain into the ostomy appliance.

42. C: The healing ridge, which is the result of collagen deposition that begins in the inflammatory stage and continues to the proliferation stage, should be evident directly under a suture line between days 5 and 9 after suturing. If the healing ridge is missing, then the wound is at increased risk of dehiscence and infection. The healing ridge appears as an area of induration extending about 1 cm on both sides of the wound.

43. C: Elbow and heel pads do not prevent pressure injuries but they do reduce friction, which can lead to skin breakdown. Friction occurs when body parts rub against the sheet or each other. Elbow pads are especially useful for patients who exhibit repetitive movements of the arms. Other methods to reduce friction include applying transparent film, skin sealant, or other protective dressings, such as a thin hydrocolloid or other padding, to vulnerable skin sites.

44. D: When cleansing a wound in a shower, the showerhead should be about 12 inches away from the wound. The showerhead may be covered with a clean washcloth or other cloth if necessary to reduce the water pressure. Showering should usually be done over 5 to 10 minutes to ensure that the wound is adequately clean. The patient may be seated in a shower chair if standing is difficult or the wound is in a hard-to-reach area.

45. A: High-level compression therapy should exert 30 to 40 mm Hg at the ankle. Low-level products exert ≤ 23 mm Hg at the ankle. Static compression utilizes various products (layered wraps, single-layer wraps, and compression stockings) to apply gradually increasing pressure to the lower extremity, distally to proximally (usually beginning at the foot or ankle and extending to the knee). The primary purpose is to prevent venous ulceration or further deterioration of existing ulcers.

46. D: Ayello's ASSESSMENTS:

A	Anatomic location and age of wound
S	Size, shape, and stage (NPIAP for pressure injury or Wagner for neurotrophic)
S	Sinus tract, tunneling, undermining, and fistulae
E	Exudate (amount, consistency, and color)
S	Sepsis

S	Surrounding skin
M	Maceration
E	Edges and epithelialization
N	Necrotic tissue
T	Tissue bed and tenderness (0-10 scale for pain)
S	Status of wound and supportive therapy

47. B: Because exposure to air will kill anaerobic bacteria, a culture should be taken with a syringe without the needle. The nurse should insert the tip of the syringe as deeply into the wound as possible, aspirating 2 to 3 mL of exudate. Immediately after removing the syringe from the wound, the nurse should attach a needle, expel all air from the syringe, and inject the exudate into a special sealed culture tube intended for anaerobic organisms. Aerobic organisms are cultured by swabbing the wound surface with a sterile swab.

48. D: BMI < 18.5. Malnutrition risk factors:

- Hypermetabolism resulting from various diseases.
- Weight loss, especially sudden or loss of 10% of normal weight over a 3-month period.
- Low body weight of < 90% of ideal body weight for age or
- Low BMI < 18.5.
- Immunosuppressive drugs that interfere with nutrient absorption, malabsorption of nutrients caused by diseases, changes in appetite, and food intolerances, such as lactose intolerance.
- Dietary restrictions, such as limiting of protein with kidney failure.
- Functional limitations such as inability to feed oneself.
- Lack of teeth or dentures, limiting intake.
- Alterations of taste or smell that render food unpalatable.

49. A: Extrinsic factors are those that derive from outside the body, such as wound bioburden. Other extrinsic factors include radiotherapy, medications, interfering therapies, and stress. Intrinsic factors are those that are inherent in the patient and can include the patient's age, disease (such as diabetes), immunosuppression (from disease, such as HIV/AIDS, or from medications, such as chemotherapeutic agents). Malnutrition and neuropathy are also intrinsic factors that can affect healing.

50. C: NPWT is intended for wounds healing by second or third intention, so the best candidate would be a stage III pressure injury. NPWT reduces edema, promotes healing, and decreases exudate but is contraindicated with exposed blood vessels, osteomyelitis, and exposed organs. For NPWT, the wound bed is filled with nonadherent porous foam and secured by occlusive transparent film into which an opening is cut over the foam and a drainage tube applied. This tube is then attached to a suction canister to create a closed system.

51. D: The clock method, which involves measuring the wound from 12 o'clock to 6 o'clock and from 9 o'clock to 3 o'clock always tracks the same site, while the GLBGW method may involve measurements at different sites each time because wounds often do not heal evenly. The clock method does require more precision to ensure that measurements are exactly perpendicular to each other. The GLBGW method is the most commonly used, but studies show it often overestimates the wound surface, while the clock method may be more accurate, but both methods can overestimate to some degree because of wound irregularities.

52. D: When testing the VPT, the nurse should first conduct a preliminary test on the patient's sternum so that the patient knows what sensation to expect. During the test, the patient should keep the eyes closed and report when first feeling a vibratory sensation and when it ceases. After striking the tuning fork, it is applied to the dorsum of the great toe (proximal to the nail bed) with the test repeated 8 times. A patient receives 1 point each time he/she fails to feel the vibration, so scores range from 0 (good) to 8 (impaired).

53. C: Immobility is the primary risk factor for development of pressure injuries, although inactivity and sensory loss are also contributing factors. People with sensory loss may not feel the discomfort that occurs with pressure. Studies have indicated that those who make 50 spontaneous movements during the night have almost no risk of developing a pressure injury, while those who make 20 or fewer spontaneous movements during the night are at high risk, highlighting the importance of frequent repositioning of patients whose mobility is limited.

54. D: Muscle tissue and granulation tissue may be similar in color; location alone is not adequate to differentiate the two. Because muscle tissue is more firm and reacts differently to pressure, the best method to differentiate the two is to palpate and gently pinch the tissue. Granulation tissue tends to be soft and spongy and will often bleed if disturbed, such as by gently pinching. Muscle tissue, however, is more resilient to pressure but may twitch if pinched or palpated.

55. A: Pulsatile lavage with suction (PLWS) is the best choice because it is effective in reducing bacterial load and can be used with undermining and tunneling. Additionally, it can be carried out effectively at bedside if necessary. Whirlpool is contraindicated in febrile patients and cannot be carried out if the patient is undergoing cardiac monitoring. Wet-to-dry dressings are no longer recommended because they may damage new tissue. Flushing a large contaminated wound with a 35 mL syringe and 19-gauge needle is likely to be ineffective.

56. B: The five Ps of neurovascular assessment are

- Pain: Amount and severity are contributing factors.
- Pallor: Indicates decreased arterial supply.
- Pulselessness: Note weak or absent pulses. Capillary refill time should be ≤ 3 seconds.
- Paresthesia: Numbness, tingling.
- Paraplegia: Assess motion.

57. B: The normal phasic flow pattern is triphasic when assessing peripheral pulses with continuous wave Doppler (representing systolic forward flow, negative deflection during diastole, and return to forward flow). As the artery loses the ability to recoil, such as through atherosclerosis, the phasic flow pattern changes to biphasic and then eventually to monophasic when the pulsatile nature of the blood flow is impaired. Continuous wave Doppler is most often used when calculating the ankle-brachial index (ABI).

58. A: The best debridement choice for a venous ulcer with hard brown adherent eschar covering 60% of the wound is autolytic with hydrogels. Because of the edema associated with venous ulcers, they tend to produce a lot of exudate, and this increases as the wound debrides, so hydrogel dressings, which have absorptive properties, help to contain the exudate and prevent maceration of the surrounding tissue. Enzymatic debridement may also be used, but the surrounding skin must be monitored carefully and protected from the enzyme and exudate.

59. D: Upon application of Apligraf to the wound, it appears similar to a skin graft. However, after about a week, it should appear gelatinous, so this is a normal transition and care must be taken not to disrupt or wash away the biological skin substitute for the first 2 to 3 weeks. In some cases, reapplication is necessary. Apligraf is supplied in a thermally controlled container and requires incubation prior to application. Apligraf is applied to the wound surface (edges overlapping) and covered with a compression wrap to secure.

60. C: Soaking dressing to loosen prior to removal relieves cyclic acute pain. CWPE model:

- Noncyclic acute wound pain: Occurs with trauma, such as sharp debridement. Interventions include topical or local anesthetics and anti-anxiety medication.
- Cyclic acute wound pain: Occurs at regular times, such as with wound changes or position changes. Interventions include soaking dressing, timeouts, nonadherent dressings, and use of repositioning devices.
- Chronic wound pain: Occurs continuously. Interventions include heat, transcutaneous nerve stimulation, and tricyclic antidepressants.

61. B: Indications of limb ischemia include ankle pressure < 40 mm Hg and toe pressure < 30 mm Hg. Critical limb ischemia occurs when resting pain is so severe it requires analgesia for more than 2 weeks of duration. Limb ischemia can result in impaired healing of arterial ulcers and increased wound pain. Pain may be evident on positional changes (increasing with elevation, decreasing with dependency), when walking (usually relieved after about 10 minutes rest), or at rest with limb elevated (neuropathic).

62. B: High-compression stockings, class IV (50–60 mmHg), are recommended only for edema associated with lymphedema, which is characterized by edema that begins soft and pitting but over time becomes firm and diffuse but more severe distally than proximally. It often occurs bilaterally and is usually not associated with pain, although the patient may complain the affected limbs feel heavy. Ulcerations are rare, and elevation provides only partial relief. Skin eventually thickens and tissue is fibrotic.

63. A: Warm mineral oil treatment for 1 week during the night can relieve dry, scaly, pruritic skin associated with peripheral edema. The legs are washed and dried thoroughly and then warm mineral oil is applied to all affected areas (usually from toes to knees). The skin is then covered with plastic wrap and secured over the feet with cotton stockings. The plastic wrap is removed in the morning and the skin washed and dried, followed by application of a thick moisturizing cream.

64. D: While all of these are attributes of foam dressings, amorphous hydrogels and alginates are used to contain wounds with a large amount of exudate. Foam dressings are highly absorbent and thermally insulating, so the primary purpose of covering these wound fillers with foam dressing is to absorb additional exudate and to raise the core temperature of the wound in order to promote autolysis. Additionally, foam dressings conform to the body and can easily mold to irregular body surfaces.

65. C: Hypertonic sodium chloride may be applied to a wound to reduce hypergranulation as it is less toxic than silver nitrate. Hypergranulation, which inhibits epithelialization, often occurs in wounds left open to heal by secondary intention. Hypertonic sodium chloride dressings are applied daily until the granulation level is normal but should be changed every 24 hours to inspect the wound. The hypertonic saline in the dressing draws excess fluid from the cells on the wound surface.

66. B: Hydrocolloids or film dressings are the best choices to provide protection to reddened skin and prevent further skin deterioration as they reduce friction and shear. Foam dressings are used for moist wounds with exudate. Sheet hydrogel is used to rehydrate slough to aide in autolysis, so it is useful when slough is present with minimal exudate. Silver dressings have antibacterial properties and are used to treat infected wounds or, as in the case of burns, to prevent infection.

67. A: 3 to 5 minutes. Procedure for lidocaine soak:

- Draw 5 to 10 mL of 2% lidocaine into a syringe.
- Remove wound dressing and cleanse wound.
- Place clean dry gauze over surface of wound.
- Saturate the wound area (and gauze) with the 2% lidocaine.
- Allow the lidocaine solution to contact the wound for 3 to 5 minutes.
- Evaluate pain sensation to ensure the area is anesthetized.
- Debride wound and redress as appropriate.

68. B: Wounds that take fewer than 14 days to heal are often partial-thickness wounds that heal with no or minimal scarring, but the potential for scarring is greater for those that take more than 14 days. Pressure dressings or garments are used commonly with burns, and special pressure garments in various sizes are available for different parts of the body. In small areas, such as on a forearm, pressure dressings may be applied with self-adherent stretch wrap or tubular dressings.

69. C: When exercising and stretching a scar, maximal stretch is usually indicated by blanching of the scar. While some pain is often involved in stretching, it should not exceed the patient's tolerance. Slow stretching that is sustained is better than rapid stretching and relaxing exercises. Exercises to stretch scars should be individually determined and depend on the type of scar, location of scar, and phase of healing, as well as patient factors, such as age, mobility, cognition, and medical status.

70. D: Signs of inflammation are usually evident in the acute surgical wound for the first 4 days, and this is a normal finding. Indications can include increased skin temperature about the incision, erythema, and edema. If no evidence of inflammation occurs, then this may indicate immunosuppression. Because hair follicles are usually present, epithelium resurfaces the incision within 72 hours, providing protection from bacteria and mild trauma, although the tensile strength of the healing incision remains weak.

71. D: High risk (90% to 100%) The Braden scale rates 5 areas (sensory perception, moisture, activity, mobility, and usual nutrition pattern) with a 1-4 scale and one area (friction and shear) with a 1-3 scale. Lower scores indicate increased risk. The scores for all six items are totaled and a risk is assigned according to the number:

- 23 (best score) = excellent prognosis, very minimal risk
- 15 to 18 = mild risk (50%-60%) with 16 usually the breakpoint for pressure injury.
- 13 to 14 = moderate risk (65%-90%).
- 10 to 12 = high risk (90%-100%) with 6 the worst score.

72. D: Pillows are useful for reducing tissue compression, especially to protect the heels, even when using support surfaces. Pillow bridging usually requires placement of at least 5 pillows with one in each of the following positions: under the legs (to protect the heels), between the ankles, between the knees, behind the back, and underneath the head. An additional small pillow may be used to support the upper arm when the patient is lying in a side-lying tilt.

73. C: Venous refill time: The procedure begins with asking the patient to lie supine for a few moments and then having the patient elevate the legs to 45 degrees for 1 minute. Next, the patient is assisted into sitting position with the feet dependent while the nurse closely observes the veins on the dorsum of the foot and counts the seconds before normal filling. Normal venous refill time is 5 to 15 seconds, and venous occlusion is indicated with times > 20 seconds.

74. A: Because these findings (swelling, drainage, pain, and purple color) are consistent with wet gangrene, no debridement should be carried out. The patient should be referred to a surgeon immediately. Wet gangrene involves necrosis of tissue from excessive moisture and bacterial infection, causing bacterial gases to accumulate in the damaged tissue. Dry gangrene occurs from impaired circulation, resulting in dry, black, shriveled tissue.

75. C: The Harris mat, used for pressure testing, is a tool that indicates the patient's plantar pressure and weight distribution and can be used to provide a pattern for off-loading. The mat is placed on the floor and opened and ink applied with a roller to the impression side. Then a piece of paper is placed on the opposite side and the impression side folded over to cover the paper (ink side down). Then, the patient steps onto the impression side and the ink transfers onto the paper with darker areas indicating areas of higher pressure.

76. D: Patients with peripheral neuropathy should have professional skin and nail care of the foot at least monthly so that the foot can be thoroughly examined and assessed in order to prevent ulceration. Those with poor hygiene or compromised tissue may need care more frequently. Toenails grow at the rate of about 1 mm per month while fingernails grow at the rate of about 3 mm per month. Toenails should be cut straight across with sharp corners smoothed with a file. Patients should be taught proper hygiene and care of the feet.

77. A: The best emollient to apply to the feet for a patient with peripheral neuropathy is petrolatum jelly because it has low water content and provides good moisturizing. Zinc oxide is used for barrier protection but is too thick for emollient purposes. Vicks VapoRub is used to soften calluses but not for routine foot care. Lotion has high water content and must be reapplied every few hours. Before application of petrolatum jelly, the feet should be washed (not soaked) with nondrying soap and dried thoroughly with clean cotton socks worn after application.

78. C: Tinea pedis (athlete's foot) is a fungal infection that can occur in those who are immunocompromised or taking broad-spectrum antibiotics. Symptoms include:

- Severe itching with vesicles or erosion of instep and with peeling maceration and fissures between toes.
- Dry, scaly, mildly erythematous patches on plantar and lateral foot surfaces.

Treatment includes selenium sulfide shampoo wash of area before applying topical antifungal (clotrimazole, miconazole, tolnaftate, naftifine, terbinafine) 2 times daily for about 4 weeks. Lambs wool may be used between toes to absorb moisture.

79. D: Electrical stimulation has been found to promote healing in most types of acute and chronic wounds and at all phases; however, ES is not recommended for children younger than 3 years, although it may be appropriate for older children. ES is also contraindicated with neoplastic wounds and evidence of osteomyelitis. If wounds penetrate to the bone, then a presumption of osteomyelitis should be made and ES avoided. Any topical treatments containing metal ions, such as povidone iodine and silver sulfadiazine, must be removed completely before ES treatment.

80. A: $TcPO_2$ level < 20 mm Hg usually indicates that a wound will not heal because oxygen supply is inadequate while a level > 30 mm Hg indicates good potential for healing, and the wound can be safely debrided. The transcutaneous method is contraindicated if edema or infection is present in the wound because results will not be accurate. Depending on the type of machine for testing, the $TcPO_2$ can take up to 30 minutes to complete.

Ostomy Care Practice Questions

1. Which of the following is the *MOST* important to determine when conducting a preoperative assessment of patient scheduled for an ostomy?

a. state of mind
b. ability to do self-care
c. family and community support
d. economic status

2. Which of the following is *MOST* likely to promote cooperation in a 25-year-old woman who required an ileostomy but refuses to look at the stoma or participate in care postoperatively?

a. refer patient to a psychologist
b. ask family to intervene
c. arrange visit with a recovered ostomate
d. advise patient of the importance of self-care

3. Which of the following is the surveillance method of choice for adolescents with familial adenomatous polyposis?

a. barium enema
b. CT scan
c. MRI
d. colonoscopy

4. How much time should elapse after placement of a percutaneous endoscopic gastrostomy (PEG) tube before the tube is secured to the abdomen?

a. 24 hours
b. until fully healed
c. 1 to 2 weeks
d. 3 to 4 days

5. Considering placement of a permanent colostomy, the anatomical position that is MOST likely to result in semi-soft, mushy stool is

a. ascending colon.
b. transverse colon.
c. descending.
d. sigmoid.

6. If a PEG tube is dislodged and pulled out 3 days after placement, the tube must be

a. replaced endoscopically.
b. replaced with a button gastrostomy.
c. replaced through the tract with a balloon gastrostomy.
d. replaced endoscopically and resited.

7. The type of drain that is flat in appearance and often placed in surgical wounds to drain fluid by gravity and capillary action is

a. simple drain.
b. sump drain.
c. closed drainage system.
d. Penrose drain.

8. The *MOST* likely anomaly in a female neonate found to have an imperforate anus with no external opening or dimple on initial physical exam, a slightly distended abdomen, and passage of some meconium at 24 hours is

a. low anomaly with rectourethral fistula.
b. intermediate anomaly with a perineal fistula.
c. high anomaly with rectovaginal fistula.
d. atypical anomaly.

9. How long after PEG is performed is the tract usually mature and healed enough for placement of a balloon gastrostomy (G-tube)?

a. 2 to 4 weeks
b. 4 to 7 days
c. 1 to 2 months
d. 3 to 4 months

10. The button gastrostomy tube may be especially recommended for

a. elderly patients.
b. bedridden patients.
c. ambulatory patients.
d. confused patients who pull on tubes.

11. What is the procedure of choice for a patient with severe intractable ulcerative colitis whose rectum remains relatively free of the disease and the anal sphincter is intact?

a. total colectomy with ileostomy
b. continent ileostomy
c. ileal pouch-anal anastomosis
d. intestinal transplant

12. A patient with regional enteritis (Crohn disease) usually has localized pain in the

a. RUQ
b. RLQ
c. LUQ
d. LLQ

13. After a colostomy, which of the following foods should generally be avoided?

a. nuts, seeds
b. apples, oranges
c. broccoli, cauliflower
d. grapes, bananas

14. Patients undergoing ostomy surgery are especially at risk for which electrolyte imbalances?

a. hypernatremia and hyperkalemia
b. hypercalcemia and hyperphosphatemia
c. hypocalcemia and hypophosphatemia
d. hyponatremia and hypokalemia

15. When marking the abdomen for placement of a stoma (excluding colostomy), the ideal site is in which muscle?

a. rectus abdominis
b. transversus abdominus
c. external oblique
d. internal oblique

16. A patient who is concerned about the copious amount of postoperative drainage from an ileostomy should be advised that

a. the amount of drainage may vary widely from one day to another.
b. the amount of drainage will decrease over time.
c. the amount of drainage may increase when the patient resumes a normal diet.
d. the amount of drainage will remain about the same.

17. What is the correct response if, in the initial period after surgery for a colostomy, the stoma appears dull and blue-tinged?

a. observe for further changes
b. notify the physician
c. no response needed, as this is normal finding
d. provide patient with nasal oxygen

18. A defunctionalized bladder remaining after urinary diversion is especially at risk for

a. pyocystis.
b. rupture.
c. prolapse.
d. fistula formation.

19. Which of the following patients is a candidate for a convex skin barrier?

a. a patient whose stoma protrudes 2 cm
b. a patient whose stoma is in the RLQ
c. a patient whose stoma protrudes 4 cm
d. a patient with a very soft pendulous abdomen

20. Stomal retraction postoperatively increases risk of

a. infection.
b. small bowel obstruction.
c. stomal stenosis.
d. stomal fistula.

21. A patient who develops stomal prolapse has a significant risk of developing

a. stomal stenosis.
b. stomal varices.
c. wound infection.
d. parastomal hernia.

22. After cleansing the PEG tube, what is the next step in rotating the tube?

a. pull the tube gently away from the abdomen 1 to 2 cm
b. gently insert the tube into the abdomen 1 to 2 cm
c. turn the tube 180° in one direction and then 180° in the other
d. turn the tube 360°

23. Which of the following complies with the American Medical Association guidelines for informed consent?

a. a patient with an inflammatory bowel disease is provided a list of treatment options
b. a patient with regional enteritis is told that her only option is a standard ileostomy
c. a preoperative patient is advised she has nothing to worry about as ostomy surgery poses little risk
d. information about a patient's condition is withheld to prevent causing her anxiety

24. Which procedure is MOST often indicated for a patient with diverticulitis, perforated diverticulum, and peritonitis?

a. end colostomy (temporary) and Hartmann's pouch
b. loop colostomy (temporary)
c. loop ileostomy (temporary)
d. colectomy

25. What advice should a woman with ulcerative colitis receive if she wants to have children and is considering having an ileal pouch-anal anastomosis (IPAA)?

a. the IPAA will not interfere with fertility or pregnancy
b. the woman should try to get pregnant prior to the IPAA
c. the woman should have the IPAA before trying to get pregnant
d. the woman cannot carry a child after having the IPAA.

26. When applying a drainage appliance for an ileostomy or colostomy, how much clearance should be allowed around the stoma?

a. 10 mm
b. 8 mm
c. 5 mm
d. 3 mm

27. Which is the MOST appropriate action to take with a patient who has undergone emergency ileostomy for Crohn's disease and severe hemorrhage but is refusing transfusions for religious reasons?

a. provide the patient with facts about the disease, treatments, and prognosis
b. ask family members to intervene
c. remind the patient that he may die without treatment
d. refer to a psychologist

28. When irrigating a Koch pouch to improve drainage postoperatively, how much maximum fluid should be instilled at one time?

a. ≤ 1000 mL
b. ≤ 500 mL
c. ≤ 100 mL
d. ≤ 40 mL

29. A patient with a high-output enterocutaneous fistula of the proximal ileum with 96 cm of small intestine remaining before the fistula would initially receive nutrition by which method?

a. oral only
b. enteral feeding
c. total parenteral nutrition
d. combination of oral and enteral

30. Which of the following procedures may result in inadequate absorption of birth control pills?

a. transverse colostomy
b. ileostomy
c. urostomy
d. descending colostomy

31. A male patient who is to have his bladder and prostate removed and is concerned about sexual functioning should be advised that

a. he will be able to ejaculate and experience orgasm.
b. he may have erectile dysfunction and will experience dry orgasm.
c. he should experience no increased sexual problems.
d. he should have no problem with erection but will experience dry orgasm.

32. What is the *BEST* explanation for a patient who complains that the gas filter on her ostomy appliance does not appear to work after she goes swimming?

a. contact with water inactivates the gas filter
b. the gas filter must be thoroughly dried after the patient goes swimming
c. contact with water should not be the cause of the problem
d. the water pressure may have damaged the filter

33. Which of the following is an initial appropriate intervention for a patient with a descending colostomy that expels softly formed stools but has persistent pancaking?

a. provide a daily laxative
b. change the appliance immediately after passing any stool
c. increase fiber in the diet
d. apply foam blocks to the inside of the pouch

34. A male ostomate with a very hairy abdomen should be advised to

a. use a chemical depilatory agent to remove hair
b. use an electric razor to remove hair once weekly
c. use a safety razor to remove hair with each appliance change
d. use extra sealant before applying an appliance

35. The most common cause of dermatitis in the peristomal area is

a. too frequent changing of appliances.
b. too infrequent changing of appliances.
c. allergic response to appliance.
d. incorrect sizing.

36. The most important factor in controlling the expelling of gas from a colostomy is

a. diet modification.
b. medication control.
c. lifestyle modification.
d. maintaining adequate fluid balance.

37. Which of the following factors is the greatest barrier to self-care?

a. age
b. hearing deficit
c. economic instability
d. cognitive impairment

38. What is the *MOST* likely cause when a patient with an ileoanal pouch develops a sudden increase in the frequency of stools as well as bloody diarrhea, fever, and fecal incontinence?

a. peritonitis
b. pouchitis
c. anastomotic lea.
d. fistula formation

39. Which of the following *MOST* indicates that a premature infant with necrotizing enterocolitis has suffered a perforation of the intestine and requires surgical intervention?

a. pneumoperitoneum
b. increased white blood cell count
c. hypoglycemia
d. feeding intolerance

40. What is the *BEST* solution for an ileostomy patient who had routinely taken enteric-coated and timed-release medications prior to surgery?

a. continue to take medications as before
b. crush the medications and mix with liquid
c. request a change in prescription to different medications
d. seek the advice of a pharmacist regarding each medication

41. Prior to surgery to create an orthotopic neobladder, the patient should be advised to

a. practice general strengthening exercises.
b. avoid heavy lifting.
c. increase fluid intake.
d. practice pelvic floor exercises.

42. Early obstruction of a colostomy stoma after surgery is *MOST* often caused by

a. edema of the bowel.
b. adhesions.
c. recurrent disease.
d. parastomal hernia.

43. Patients with which type of ostomy are *MOST* likely to benefit from routine ostomy irrigations to control fecal output?

a. ileostomy
b. ascending colostomy
c. descending colostomy
d. transverse colostomy

44. What intervention is advised for a patient to relieve cramping following a colostomy irrigation?

a. gently massaging the abdomen
b. walking
c. taking an antacid
d. drinking warm liquid

45. Patients with familial adenomatous polyposis (FAP) should be monitored routinely for which extracolonic cancer?

a. lung
b. thyroid
c. ovarian
d. pancreas

46. A porridge (oatmeal) enema test can be used to

a. evaluate sphincter function and potential for fecal continence.
b. facilitate bowel training after reanastomosis.
c. evaluate peristaltic action in the distal portion of the bowel.
d. evaluate stoma strictures.

47. In order to avoid an ostomy in an infant with bladder exstrophy, surgical repair of the bladder should be done within

a. 24 hours.
b. 72 hours.
c. 1 week.
d. 2 weeks.

48. The ureteral stents in place after a urostomy are usually left in place for

a. 24 hours.
b. 5 to 14 days.
c. 48 to 72 hours.
d. 3 to 4 weeks.

49. How would a patient be positioned for an endoanal ultrasound?

a. prone
b. supine with legs in stirrups
c. left side-lying
d. right side-lying

50. Which of the following conditions is usually a contraindication for IPAA?

a. colon cancer
b. regional enteritis (Crohn's disease)
c. familial adenomatous polyposis (FAP)
d. ulcerative colitis

51. Which test is indicated to evaluate a possible anastomotic leak from an IPAA?

a. CT scan
b. defecating pouchogram
c. MRI
d. radiograph

52. When assessing factors that affect readiness to learn, a patient's cultural background and personal goals relate to which of the following?

a. physical factors
b. mental/emotional status
c. experience
d. knowledge/education

53. What is the appropriate intervention for an ostomate who is receiving chemotherapy and develops a small sore and increased bleeding of the stoma?

a. cauterize sore with silver nitrate
b. flush stoma area with antibiotic solution
c. apply topical corticosteroid to stoma
d. do gentle routine care

54. What dressing strategy is usually used for low-output fistulas?

a. skin barrier and absorptive dressings
b. alginate and secondary dressings
c. solid skin barrier and ostomy appliance
d. gauze dressing only.

55. The most common cause of spontaneous enterocutaneous fistula is

a. Crohn's disease.
b. diverticulosis.
c. ulcerative colitis.
d. colon cancer.

56. If a patient with a J-PEG (jejunostomy) tube develops vomiting, Abdominal distension, and increasing abdominal pain, the nurse should suspect

a. perforation.
b. blockage.
c. migration.
d. breakage.

57. Following formation of an orthotopic neobladder, how frequently should patients generally schedule urination in the first week after the catheter is removed?

a. every 2 hours during the daytime and every 3 hours at night
b. every 3 hours during the daytime and every 4 hours at night
c. every 4 hours during the daytime and every 5 hours at night
d. every 5 hours during the daytime and every 6 hours at night

58. If urine does not flow freely or at all during routine catheterization of a continent urinary diversion, the patient should

a. remove the catheter.
b. insert the catheter a few centimeters further into the pouch.
c. irrigate the catheter.
d. stand and walk around before removing catheter.

59. Which is the best solution for a patient who complains of skin irritation and odor from the mucous fistula that formed when she had an emergency ileostomy?

a. change the gauze dressings more frequently
b. use a skin barrier and deodorizing stoma bag or cap
c. apply odor eliminator drops (such as M9) to the gauze dressing
d. apply gauze dressing and cover with waterproof tape to contain odor

60. Compared with continent cutaneus urinary diversion, the orthotopic neobladder has significantly increased incidence of

a. urinary obstruction.
b. parastomal hernia.
c. urinary infection.
d. wound complications.

61. Patients with bladder cancer that has invaded multiple areas of the bladder muscle are usually treated with

a. radiation alone.
b. segmental cystectomy.
c. radical cystectomy and urinary diversion.
d. chemotherapy alone.

62. For a male patient doing clean intermittent catheterization, which type of tip is best if the patient has a urethral stricture?

a. straight
b. coudé
c. olive tipped
d. personal preference

63. The most likely consequence of an orthotopic neobladder created from an ileocecal resection is

a. vitamin B12 deficiency.
b. decreased storage capacity.
c. diarrhea.
d. increased frequency of stools and risk of steatorrhea.

64. When draining an ileostomy pouch into a toilet, what can the patient do to avoid splashing stool and water?

a. sit further away from the toilet
b. place sheets of toilet tissue on the water in the toilet bowl
c. partially open the pouch
d. put the end of the pouch into the water

65. Which dressing choice is *MOST* practical for the stoma of a continent cutaneous fecal diversion?

a. barrier wafer and stoma appliance
b. no dressing is necessary
c. stoma cap
d. gauze pad

66. A fistula that drains yellow/orange fluid usually originates in the

a. stomach.
b. duodenum.
c. small intestine.
d. colon.

67. What is the earliest that reversal of a colostomy or ileostomy can usually be safely performed?

a. 1 month
b. 2 months
c. 6 months
d. 8 months

68. What is the medication of choice for the treatment of mild ulcerative colitis?

a. mesalazine
b. sulfasalazine
c. budesonide
d. infliximab

69. Patients with spina bifida are at high risk for which of the following?

a. intellectual disability.
b. underweight.
c. latex allergy.
d. diabetes mellitus type 1.

70. A patient undergoing an abdominoperineal resection of the rectum (APER) should expect which of the following to be resected?

a. the rectum and the anal canal.
b. the rectum.
c. the rectum, part of the sigmoid colon, and the anal canal.
d. the rectum, part of the sigmoid colon, the anal canal, and anal sphincters

71. What does it indicate if a patient with severe cognitive impairment underwent emergency formation of a colostomy and is receiving pain medication around the clock but has short periods of hyperventilation, cries out frequently, is lying rigidly with fists clenched, and is increasingly combative?

a. inadequate pain control
b. excess sedation from pain medication
c. side effects of pain medication
d. increasing dementia

72. How often are urostomy appliances usually emptied?

a. 2 times daily
b. 3 to 4 times daily
c. 4 to 6 times daily
d. 8 to 10 times daily

73. Which of the following is a common complication after takedown of a loop ileostomy?

a. dehiscence
b. small bowel obstruction
c. hemorrhage
d. chronic pain

74. What is the primary cause of chronic or recurrent perianal irritation after IPAA?

a. poor hygiene
b. digestive acids and enzymes
c. improper food choices
d. medications

75. Malabsorption of bile salts may result in

a. decreased bowel frequency.
b. pouchitis.
c. increased bowel frequency.
d. obstruction.

76. How much fluid should a patient with an ileostomy be advised to drink each day?

a. 800 mL
b. 1000 mL
c. 1500 mL
d. 2000 mL

77. How frequently should a patient with an orthotopic neobladder and the ability to urinate well do a routine catheterization?

a. daily
b. weekly
c. monthly
d. when problems arise

78. The ideal protrusion of an ileostomy stoma is

a. none, the stoma should be flush.
b. 0.5 cm
c. 2 cm.
d. 3 cm.

79. What is the BEST solution for a patient who has had his colon and rectum removed but complains of rectal pressure and the sensation of needing to defecate?

a. relaxation exercises
b. sitting on the toilet and bearing down as though defecating
c. biofeedback
d. analgesia

80. What is the initial intervention for a dietary obstruction of an IPAA?

a. laxative
b. irrigation
c. liquids only for 24 hours
d. high-residue diet

Ostomy Care Answers and Explanations

1. B: While all of these are important aspects to evaluate, the patient's ability to do self-care is primary because this can help determine the type of procedure that is best for the patient as well as the extent and type of postoperative care and education that may be needed. If the patient is not able to manage self-care, then the presence and abilities of caregivers must be evaluated as well. Low economic status may affect the patient's ability to purchase needed supplies and to manage care.

2. C: A visit from a recovered ostomate who is functioning well can provide invaluable support. Refusing to look at the stoma or participate in care after surgery is very common as patients grapple with the alteration in body image and anxiety about their role in family and society, their sexuality, and their ability to resume their normal activities. Family members should be encouraged to learn about ostomy care and to provide support as well, but they may also be very stressed and unsure. Referral to a psychologist may be indicated if the patient cannot overcome her anxiety and fears.

3. D: Colonoscopy is the surveillance method of choice for FAP, with routine surveillance usually beginning between 10 and 15 years, depending on the severity of the disease. Genetic testing is available to identify the type of FAP, as the rate of colorectal cancer varies somewhat. The most common genetic mutation is of the APC gene (chromosome 5q21), which carries a 75% risk of cancer by age 20 and 90% risk by age 30. Patients with high risk of colorectal cancer may be advised to have a prophylactic colectomy.

4. B: The PEG tube should not be secured to the abdomen until the PEG is fully healed because tension caused by taping the tube against the abdomen may cause the tract to change shape and direction. The tract should be straight to facilitate insertion and removal of catheters. A solid skin barrier with the tube fed through an anchored baby nipple is an inexpensive stabilizer that keeps the tube in correct position. Position and length of tube should be carefully documented.

5. C: A permanent colostomy in the descending colon is most likely to result in semi-soft, mushy stool. A colostomy in the ascending colon results in liquid stool as little absorption has taken place as liquid stool enters the colon from the small intestine. A transverse colostomy results in semi-liquid, somewhat mushy stool. Because the sigmoid colostomy is directly above the rectum, most excess fluid has been absorbed by the proximal colon, so stool tends to be more solid.

6. A: If a PEG tube is pulled out in the first 7 to 10 days after placement, the tract is not yet mature enough for a replacement catheter to be inserted through the tract, so the PEG must be replaced endoscopically. The replacement should be carried out as soon as possible because the tract will begin to close within a few hours. Resiting of the tube should not be necessary unless there is extensive trauma for some reason.

7. D: The Penrose drain is a soft, flat rubber/latex tubes placed in surgical wounds to drain fluid by gravity and capillary action. Simple drains are latex or vinyl tubes of varying sizes and lengths inserted usually into a stab wound to provide drainage of serous material, blood, pus, or other discharge. Sump drains are double-lumen or tri-lumen tubes (with a third lumen for infusions). A large outflow lumen and small inflow lumen produces venting when air enters the inflow lumen and forces drainage into the large lumen. A closed drainage system uses low-pressure suction to provide continuous gravity drainage of wounds.

8. C: Anorectal abnormalities, such as imperforate anus, result from abnormal development, and they are classified according to the rectum's relationship to puborectalis muscle. A high anomaly occurs when the rectum is positioned above the puborectalis muscle and the child lacks an internal sphincter. Most commonly, this defect is associated with a rectourethral fistula in a male child and a rectovaginal fistula in a female child. This fistula accounts for the passage of some meconium even without an external opening.

9. A: The tract of a PEG usually matures and heals within 2 to 4 weeks. Once the tract has healed, the original PEG tube can generally be replaced with a balloon gastrostomy tube. Gastrostomy tubes with an internal balloon or mushroom tip, measured markings, and an external disk are easier to stabilize, but internal devices should be checked daily by gently pulling until resistance is felt. External stabilizing devices can be applied to the skin to hold the tube in place. The tube may also be taped to the abdomen or secured with a binder.

10. D: The button gastrostomy tube, which is secured by a balloon or traction device, lies flat against the abdomen, and is often recommended for patients who are confused and pull on tubes, especially if they have already pulled out a gastrostomy tube, because it is more difficult to grasp and pull out. The button gastrostomy tube is also often recommended for younger ambulatory patients who are concerned about the external appearance of the tube and want to wear fashionable clothing.

11. C: The procedure of choice for a patient with severe intractable ulcerative colitis is IPAA if the rectum is relatively free of disease and the anal sphincter is intact. If the rectum is severely diseased, complete excision of the colon, rectum, and anus is recommended, as disease will recur. Usually after the diseased colon is removed, extraintestinal manifestations of the disease subside. Surgery is indicated when the patient continues to deteriorate and does not respond to conservative treatment.

12. B: With regional enteritis, pain is most commonly localized in the right lower quadrant. Borborygmus and increased peristalsis result in hyperactive bowel sounds noted on auscultation. Patients complain of abdominal tenderness on palpation. The most common symptom is intermittent pain, occurring with diarrhea but unrelieved by defecation. Pain usually occurs after eating because this stimulates peristalsis. If the terminal ileum is involved, pain may occur in the periumbilical area. Patients often begin to limit food intake to control pain, but this can result in malnutrition and anemia.

13. A: While individual sensitivity to foods varies, in general patients should avoid foods high in cellulose or hemicellulose, such as nuts and seeds, because they retain fluid and stimulate peristalsis and may also cause obstruction. Some foods should be eaten in moderation, including fruits such as prunes, grapes, and bananas. Cruciferous vegetables, such as broccoli and cauliflower, may increase gas and odor. Patients should be advised to keep a food diary to help to determine which foods are most irritating to them.

14. D: The primary electrolyte regulating fluid balance is sodium, which works in conjunction with potassium, so excess fluid loss, common in ostomy patients, can result in hyponatremia and hypokalemia. Symptoms of hyponatremia include irritability, lethargy, and alterations in consciousness; cerebral edema with seizures and coma; and dyspnea leading to respiratory failure. Symptoms of hypokalemia include lethargy and weakness, hypotension, nausea and vomiting, paresthesia, muscle cramps with hyporeflexia, dysrhythmias with ECG abnormalities such as premature ventricular contractions and flattened T waves.

15. A: Ideally, the stoma should be placed in the rectus abdominis muscle, which stretches from the rib cage to the pelvis. In most cases (excluding colostomy), the best placement is in the RLQ about 2 inches (10 cm) below the waist so the person's belt and bending motions do not interfere with the stoma; however, this placement may not always be possible. The stoma should not be placed in folds or scar tissue and should be easily accessible by the patient.

16. B: In the immediate postoperative period, drainage from an ileostomy may be up to about 1800 mL/day. Initially, the drainage may be thick and greenish but it then becomes watery with constant drainage because the small intestine usually reabsorbs little fluid; however, as time passes, the small bowel begins to compensate for the lack of the colon and absorbs more fluid, decreasing the output to about 500 to 800 mL/day and thickening the stool.

17. B: While the stoma may be edematous in the initial postoperative period, it should appear red to pink, shiny, and moist, indicating adequate oxygenation and healthy tissue. If the stoma appears dull and cyanotic (blue to purple to brown/black if the tissue becomes necrotic), the physician should be notified immediately because reoperation to increase blood flow to the tissue may be indicated. The stoma should be assessed for circulatory impairment on a regular schedule after surgery.

18. A: While a cystectomy is usually performed as part of urinary diversion procedures, in some cases, the bladder is left in place. Because the mucous lining of the bladder still secretes, discharge can build up in the defunctionalized bladder. Usually, these secretions are expelled periodically, but if blockage occurs, the secretions continue to collect in the bladder and may become infected, resulting in pyocystis. Treatment of pyocystis usually includes drainage and antibiotics.

19. D: Convex skin barriers help to create a tight seal around stomas that are flush or retracted, but they are also appropriate to use with a patient with a very soft pendulous abdomen or where folds in the skin interfere with the appliance. Appliances are available with shallow, moderate, and deep convexity, but a barrier ring, with adhesive on both sides, can be placed around the stoma to create convexity as well if only flat skin barrier wafers are available.

20. C: Stomal retraction, usually caused by increased tension on the intestine or stoma, is associated with increased risk of stenosis, especially if the retraction results from ischemia. Mild stomal retraction is managed with convex skin barriers, but if the retraction is severe, local repair and creation of a new stoma are indicated. If stenosis is present, then the scar tissue may need to be excised because attempting to dilate the stenotic area may increase the stenosis.

21. D: About half of the patients who develop a significant stomal prolapse also develop a parastomal hernia. Obese patients and those with COPD are at increased risk of developing stomal prolapse, but is may also occur with inadequate surgical construction or creation of a stoma outside of the rectus abdominis. Prolapse may be fixed or a sliding stoma prolapse, which is more likely to develop incarceration. The prolapsed portion may be repaired with resection and surgical stapling.

22. B: When rotating the PEG tube, an important step in preventing adherence and promoting healing of the tract, the tube should be gently inserted 1 to 2 cm so that the internal stabilizing device is pushed away from the tissue so that rotation does not cause trauma. Then, the tube is slowly turned 360°. Next, the tube is gently pulled back out until the interior stabilizing device is in correct position and the external stabilizing device secured.

23. A: The patient with inflammatory bowel disease is provided a list of possible treatment options, as required by the guidelines for informed consent. Surgical repair for regional enteritis is done in different ways, so providing one option limits the patient's right to choose. Telling a patient she has nothing to worry about is a platitude and may be wrong. Patients have a legal right to information about their conditions, even if it may cause anxiety. Patients cannot make informed consent without adequate and accurate information.

24. A: The procedure usually performed for a patient with diverticulitis, perforated diverticulum, and peritonitis is the end colostomy (temporary) and Hartmann's pouch. The affected parts of the colon (often the sigmoid and part of the descending colon) are removed surgically, but anastomosis must be delayed until the infection clears, so a Hartmann pouch with the intact rectum is left in place so that the colostomy can be removed at a later time and reanastomosis completed.

25. B: While women have successfully carried pregnancies after IPAA, the ileoanal pouch has been associated with about a 50% drop in fertility, so the woman should be advised to try to get pregnant and complete childbearing prior to having the IPAA. There is not yet consensus about the best method of delivery, although there seems to be increased risk with vaginal delivery, especially if tearing of the anal sphincter occurs. Most women are advised to have cesarean deliveries.

26. D: When applying a drainage appliance for an ileostomy or colostomy, about 3 mm clearance should be allowed around the stoma. Exposed skin may become macerated, so a skin barrier should be applied under to the exposed skin. The appliance should fit snugly about the stoma but not so tightly that it could cause trauma. The size of the stoma may vary from time to time, so this must be considered when fitting an appliance.

27. A: Patients have a right to refuse treatment for religious or other personal reasons, so the most appropriate action is to simply provide the patient with factual information about the blood loss and prognosis in a neutral manner, without trying to coerce or frighten the patient. In some cases, patients may change their minds when presented with information, but the nurse should remain supportive regardless of the patient's decision. Asking the family to intervene is not appropriate, and refusal of treatment alone does not suggest the need for referral to a psychologist.

28. D: The Koch pouch may need to be irrigated postoperatively to promote drainage because of the accumulation of mucus. Also, once the patient begins to eat, drainage may slow, requiring irrigation. Up to 1000 mL of total of solution (usually tap water) may be needed to flush the pouch but only 30 to 40 mL of fluid should be instilled at one time as the capacity of the pouch is small. The instilled fluid should be drained completely before doing another instillation and the patient observed carefully for abdominal discomfort.

29. C: A patient with a small amount of small intestine (less than 100 cm) before the fistula and high-output fistula usually is kept NPO initially because eating stimulates increased loss of fluids, resulting in increased electrolyte imbalance, and protein, leading to increased malnutrition. Enteral feeding is commonly used for fistula affecting the duodenum, distal ileum, or colon. Patients able to maintain adequate oral intake should eat a diet high in calorie and sodium but low in fiber, which may cause fistula blockage.

30. B: Women of childbearing age with an ileostomy should be advised that absorption of birth control pills may be impaired because the medication is generally absorbed in the small intestine. Thus, they may want to consider other options such as an IUD or diaphragm for birth control, but they should discuss use of these devices with health care professionals if part of the vaginal wall or the rectum has been removed. Women with urostomy, transverse, descending, or sigmoid colostomies generally should be able to take birth control pills without concerns about absorption.

31. B: When discussing sexual issues, the patient should be provided complete and honest information. Following removal of the prostate and bladder, the male patient often experiences erectile dysfunction and will not be able to ejaculate but can achieve a dry orgasm. Interventions to help the patient achieve an erection will vary depending on whether he has partial or complete nerve damage or other problems, such as anxiety, that are preventing erection.

32. A: Gas (flatus) filters are inactivated if they come in contact with water, so the patient wearing the appliance in the bath or while swimming should apply a waterproof cover (usually supplied by the manufacturer) or cover with a strip of waterproof tape. Filters contain carbon to neutralize odors and must control for sulfurous and complex organic odors, so patients may need to experiment to determine which type of filter is most effective for them.

33. D: While dietary modifications are sometimes indicated to help control pancaking, the patient's stool is soft and formed already, so the best initial intervention is to apply foam blocks or other bridging device to the inside of the pouch to prevent the two sides of the appliance from adhering. Other solutions include applying oil to the inside of the appliance or special lubricating gels. Some people remove the flatus filters, but this may result in ballooning.

34. B: Hair can interfere with appliance adherence, even with the use of sealants, so the best method is to shave with an electric razor. Depilatories should be avoided as they may irritate the skin, and small nicks may occur with a safety razor. Inflammation of the hair follicles (folliculitis) may occur in those with abdominal hair because of irritation from application and removal of appliances or from too frequent shaving, so shaving should be done no more frequently than once a week.

35. D: While some people have allergic responses to the sealant or appliance, the most common cause of dermatitis in the peristomal area is incorrect sizing that leaves too much skin exposed around the stoma, increasing the risk of leakage under the appliance as well as irritation of the exposed skin. Patients should be advised to measure their stomas with each appliance change for at least 6 to 8 weeks after surgery until the stoma size stabilizes and then periodically. The stoma opening should not be more than 3 mm larger than the stoma size.

36. A: The most important factor in controlling the expelling of gas from a colostomy is diet modification, and this can include modifying both the types of foods in the diet as well as the manner of eating and drinking. Patients should chew food slowly and completely and avoid talking while eating. They may also benefit from small frequent meals rather than 3 large meals daily. Patients should avoid drinking fluids through straws and avoid carbonated drinks. Reducing fiber and avoiding cruciferous vegetables, nonabsorbable sugars, and resistant starches may also help.

37. D: While all of these may pose a challenge, cognitive impairment poses the greatest barrier to self-care because instruction may need to be repeated many times and steps to managing an ostomy broken down into simple steps. Picture guides, or in some cases written guides, may also be helpful, depending on the patient's degree of cognitive impairment. If cognitive impairment is profound, such as with advanced Alzheimer disease, then self-care may not be a realistic goal.

38. B: Increased frequency of stools, bloody diarrhea, fever, and fecal incontinence are signs of pouchitis, nonspecific inflammation of the pouch. Although the cause is not known, pouchitis may indicate undiagnosed regional enteritis (Crohn disease) in some patients, although it is more common in patients with ulcerative colitis. Pouchitis is most common in the first 2 years after surgery. Pouchitis usually responds rapidly to metronidazole, and this helps to differentiate the condition from others that may cause similar symptoms.

39. A: Pneumoperitoneum is the primary predictor that perforation or necrosis of the bowel has occurred, resulting in the need for surgical intervention. Necrotizing enterocolitis (NEC) is the most common gastrointestinal emergency in premature neonates. Seventy-five percent of neonates who develop NEC are less than 37 weeks' gestation and weigh less than 2000 grams. NEC is an acute necrosis in 1 or multiple bowel segments anywhere from the stomach to the rectum. Inflammation occurs, and often bacterial invasion, and perforation. Initial treatment is NG decompression, IV fluids, and antibiotics.

40. D: While enteric-coated and timed-release medications may not be properly absorbed if left intact because the part of the bowel that normally absorbs the medication is missing, some medications may be inactivated by stomach acids, so each medication should be discussed with a pharmacist to determine if crushing the medication and mixing it with liquids is acceptable. In some cases, different medications or different doses may be necessary, and the pharmacist is best able to discuss alternatives.

41. D: Both before and after surgery for creation of an orthotopic neobladder, male and female patients should be advised to practice pelvic floor (Kegel) exercises to strengthen the sphincter muscles. Patients should do exercises sitting, standing, and lying supine at least twice daily and should try to complete at least 40 cycles of contracting and holding and 40 of quick contractions. After surgery, patients should increase exercises in positions in which they have the most leakage, such as when lying supine at night.

42. A: Early obstruction of a colostomy stoma after surgery is most often caused by edema of the bowel or technical problems with the surgery. Once the patient starts to eat, obstruction may also occur with a bolus of food, so foods should be introduced slowly to the diet. Obstruction related to adhesions, recurrent disease (especially Crohn's disease), and parastomal hernia are usually late obstructions, and do not occur in the immediate postoperative period.

43. C: Irrigations to control fecal output are generally used only for descending or sigmoid colostomies, as fecal output is too high in ascending or transverse colostomies. Irrigations are generally not advised for ileostomies. Frequency of irrigation varies, but every other day is the most common schedule. It may take about 6 weeks of routine irrigation before the bowel is regulated, so patients should be advised that the procedure requires some initial patience.

44. A: Cramping is usually relieved by gently massaging the abdomen. Some patients also find that deep breathing and relaxing also helps as the cramping may be exacerbated by tension. While walking might also relieve cramping, if the fluid has not been completely expelled already, getting up in the middle of the irrigation procedure to move around can prove messy. Cramping may result from excess fluid instillation or too-rapid instillation.

45. B: Patients with FAP have increased risk of extracolonic cancers, especially of the thyroid, so they should be monitored routinely. Additionally, other extracolonic manifestations of FAP include osteomas, epidermoid cysts, desmoid tumors, adrenal and duodenal adenomas, hepatoblastoma, abnormal dentition, and congenital hypertrophy of the retinal pigment epithelium (CHRPE). The most common cause of death in untreated FAP is colorectal cancer, but even those who have colectomy/IPAA are at risk for eventual development of duodenal adenoma.

46. A: The porridge (oatmeal) enema test is a simple method to evaluate sphincter function before stoma closure. The enema can be instilled into the distal stoma or the rectum. The oatmeal (or in some cases instant mashed potatoes) is thickened to the consistency of a normal soft stool. The patients are evaluated for fecal leakage lying down, sitting, standing, and after normal activities, including walking around, for 30 minutes. Those who can retain the enema for 30 minutes are generally good candidates for fecal continence after reanastomosis.

47. B: Treatment for bladder exstrophy:

First stage:

- Primary closure of bladder: No ostomy necessary if done within 72 hours of birth. Procedures include ureteral stents and suprapubic urinary drainage.
- Bilateral iliac ostomies: Necessary after 72 hours because pelvic ring is not malleable.
- Epispadias repair: May be done in first or second stage.

Second stage:

- Epispadias repair: Usually done between 6 and 12 months.

Final stage:

- Bladder neck reconstruction and reimplantation of ureters.
- Permanent urinary diversion: Required by 10% to 15%.

48. B: Ureteral stents are usually removed after 5 to 14 days, although they may be left in for several weeks. Each protruding stent should be drained separately and clearly labeled. Stents have multiple holes along the length of the tube to promote drainage. It is important to ensure that the stents are not dislodged or blocked. If pain, purulent discharge, or fever occurs, an x-ray may be taken to determine position of the stent. Patient must be advised NOT to remove the stent.

49. C: Endoanal ultrasound is used to diagnose perianal fistulas and abscesses and to assess sphincter damage related to fecal incontinence and for staging and follow-up of malignant infiltrations of sphincters with anal neoplasms. Procedure:

- With the patient lying on the left side, a narrow, wand-like endoscopic probe with a transducer and a lubricated rigid plastic cone covering the end is inserted into the anal canal and pictures are viewed on a computer screen. The cone has a uniform diameter to prevent anatomical distortion.
- Patients may feel vibration during procedure.

50. B: Regional enteritis (Crohn's disease) is usually a contraindication for IPAA because the failure rate with Crohn's disease is up to 60%. IPAA is primarily indicated for those with ulcerative colitis, indeterminate ulcerative colitis, or familial adenomatous polyposis. IPAA is used less frequently with colon cancer but may be indicated if the margins are clear and the cancer has not spread into the surrounding tissues. IPAA may be done at any age but patients older than 55 years may have more problems with incontinence.

51. C: The pelvic MRI is recommended to evaluate for a possible anastomotic leak from an IPAA. If a leak occurs, the patient may develop pelvic sepsis, most commonly in the early postoperative period. Symptoms may include poorly functioning pouch and pain. Symptoms are similar to those of pouchitis, so an MRI can differentiate. Anastomotic leak may require antibiotic therapy alone or surgical repair as well if a collection of fluid is found on MRI.

52. C: Experience with learning can vary widely and is affected by ability to cope with changes, personal goals, motivation to learn, and cultural background. People may have widely divergent ideas about what constitutes illness and/or treatment. Lack of English skills may make learning difficult and prevent people from asking questions. The patients' and families' readiness to learn should be assessed because if they are not ready, instruction is of little value. Often readiness is indicated when the patients/families ask questions or show an interest in procedures.

53. D: Ostomates undergoing chemotherapy often exhibit increased swelling and bleeding of the stoma as well as mouth and stoma sores. No specific treatment is indicated, as the sores will generally heal when chemotherapy stops. The stoma should be gently cleansed to decrease the chance of bleeding and pressure applied if bleeding occurs. The size of the appliance opening may need to be increased because of swelling. Some patients develop constipation because of dehydration related to nausea and vomiting, while others develop persistent diarrhea.

54. A: Low-output fistulas (less than 150 mL per 24 hours) may need only skin barriers and easily changed absorbent dressings. If drainage cannot be contained with an absorbent dressing, then ostomy appliances with solid skin barriers and pouches are indicated. The barrier should extend at least 1.5 inches around the perimeter of the fistula. The barrier must adhere to even skin to avoid drainage getting under the barrier, so the opening may need to be enlarged. Pouching systems with barriers that can be cut to fit usually work best. Very large wounds (more than 4 inches) may require a custom pouching system.

55. A: The most common cause of spontaneous enterocutaneous fistula is Crohn's disease. Most fistulae occur postoperatively but 20% to 30% occur spontaneously. Ulcerative colitis (UC) may also occasionally result in spontaneous fistula, but UC is more commonly associated with postoperative fistula. Diverticulosis rarely results in fistula except postoperatively. Other causes of spontaneous fistula include cancer, radiation, and intra-abdominal sepsis.

56. C: These symptoms are indications of J-PEG migration, which is unique to J-PEG tubes. If the J-tube migrates proximally, the patient may experience vomiting and increased risk of aspiration while if the J-tube migrates distally, the patient may experience vomiting, Abdominal distension, and increasing abdominal pain. If tube migration is suspected, then fluid should be aspirated and tested for pH using a colorimetric pH strip. The tube should be marked carefully, checked frequently, and secured to prevent migration.

57. A: After the catheter is removed following creation of a neobladder, the patient begins scheduled urination in the sitting position, usually every 2 hours during the day and every 3 hours at night. Some incontinence is normal, especially during the night. The time between scheduled urination usually increases by about 1 hour per week up until 5 weeks, when patients should be able to go 6 hours between urinations, but this may vary with individuals. Patients should be advised to not exceed 6 hours between urinations, even at night.

58. C: If urine does not flow freely or at all, this usually indicates that the catheter is blocked by mucus. While removing the catheter and flushing it may solve the immediate problem, there may be more mucus in the pouch, so the best solution is to irrigate. Irrigation is usually done with 60 mL of normal saline, which is instilled and drained, repeating this procedure until the fluid runs clear of mucus and drains freely.

59. B: Because this patient has both skin irritation and odor, the best solution is to apply a skin barrier, such as a wafer, and a deodorizing stoma bag or stoma cap, depending on the amount of drainage. The mucous fistula continues to drain mucus that forms in the distal bowel, and this may be quite malodorous, especially in the initial postoperative period. In some cases, the discharge may be quite watery. The skin around the mucous fistula should be cleansed with water and dried thoroughly with each dressing change.

60. D: The neobladder has a higher rate of wound complications (34%) than does continent urinary diversion (19%) within 5 years of surgery but both types of procedures result in numerous complications. The neobladder has 3 times the incidence of urinary stones and fistulae, although there is little difference in the rates of urinary obstruction or infection, parastomal hernias, or stoma complications. Studies indicate that patients receiving continent urinary diversion or neobladder should have long-term monitoring for complications.

61. C: The most common treatment for invasive bladder cancer is radical cystectomy and urinary diversion, although some patients may undergo radiation and chemotherapy in addition to or in place of surgery, depending on the stage and extent of the cancer. Urinary diversion includes urostomy, continent cutaneous urinary diversion with a pouch formed from part of the bowel and an external stoma that must be catheterized, and orthotopic neobladder, which allows urination through the urethra. Segmental cystectomy is generally restricted to those whose cancer is low grade and whose disease has affected only one area of the bladder.

62. B: The Coudé curved-tip intermittent-use catheter is often used for men with urethral strictures or enlarged prostates to facilitate catheterization as the tip of the catheter is quite small. The straight catheter is most commonly used by women and many men as well. The olive-tipped catheter has a guide strip and is useful for people who have difficulty with insertion. Men usually require at least a 12-inch catheter, but women and children may use a shorter and more compact catheter.

63. D: Creating an orthotopic neobladder from an ileocecal resection may result in increased frequency of stools and risk of steatorrhea. These patients are also at increased risk of developing (oxalate) kidney stones and gallstones because of loss of bile acid. Ileal resection is associated with malabsorption of vitamins B12, D, E, and K with resections of more than 100 cm of bowel. Colonic/sigmoid resection may result in diarrhea because less fluid and sodium are absorbed and there is decreased storage capacity.

64. B: When liquid or semi-liquid contacts another liquid, splashing almost always occurs, but placing sheets of toilet tissue in the water in the toilet bowl often provides enough of a barrier to keep the stool from splashing. Patients usually empty their pouches while sitting on the toilet, although some may prefer to sit on a chair facing the toilet, especially if they are obese or very large. They unroll the bottom of the pouch into the toilet but should avoid contact with the water.

65. D: The stoma for a continent cutaneous fecal diversion is a small nipple valve, usually about one-half inch in diameter in the lower right quadrant of the abdomen. Unless a complication arises, the stoma should not leak stool. The most inexpensive and easiest dressing to use is a gauze square, which will absorb mucous drainage. Once the pouch is well healed and has reached its maximum size, most people are able to empty the pouch only 3 to 4 times daily.

66. C: A fistula that drains yellow/orange fluid usually originates in the small intestine. External fistulae are often first detected when drainage from a wound increases. A fistula from the stomach may drain clear, watery fluid while bile staining may occur with a fistula involving the duodenum. Brown, fecal-appearing, and odorous drainage usually occurs with fistula of the large intestine. Because of digestive enzymes found in chyme, drainage may rapidly result in skin excoriation.

67. B: Reversal of a colostomy or ileostomy should usually be done only after a minimum of 2 months because the bowel may remain edematous for that period of time, and any abnormality of the bowel increases the risk of postoperative complications. However, in many cases, reversal is done after a longer time period, such as 3 to 6 months. Reanastomosis is done by suturing or stapling the proximal and distal ends. With loop ostomies, reanastomosis may be completed without surgically opening the abdomen.

68. A: The medication of choice for mild ulcerative colitis is mesalazine, or 5-aminosalicylate (5-ASA), with the most effective dosing at least 2 g daily. This drug is used more frequently than sulfasalazine, which has more side effects. Corticosteroids, such as budesonide, are used when disease does not respond adequately to the 5-ASA medication. Steroids are more commonly used for acute disease, but if the disease does not respond adequately or if patients cannot tolerate corticosteroids, immunosuppressive drugs, such as infliximab, may be considered.

69. C: Patients with spina bifida are at high risk of latex allergy because they often must do clean intermittent catheterizations and may have multiple surgeries, all of which have the potential to expose the patient to latex, resulting in sensitization, which may progress to an anaphylactic reaction. Patients may exhibit few or only mild symptoms, such as itching, erythema, sneezing, and cough, when in contact with latex, and may not be aware that these are indications of latex allergy, so all spina bifida patients should be considered latex allergic.

70. D: A patient undergoing an abdominoperineal resection of the rectum (APER) should expect that the rectum, part of the sigmoid colon, the anal canal, and the anal sphincters will be removed, and a colostomy created, usually in the LLQ. This procedure is usually reserved for those with a tumor low in the rectum or for those with severe regional enteritis (Crohn's disease) that has not responded to more conservative medical therapy. Those with Crohn's disease treated with steroids may have delayed healing.

71. A: The patient is exhibiting nonverbal indications of pain. The Pain Assessment in Advanced Dementia (PAINAD) scale is as follows:

- Respirations: Rapid and labored breathing as pain increases, with short periods of hyperventilation or Cheyne-Stokes respirations.
- Vocalization: Negative in speech or speaking quietly and reluctantly, may moan or groan. As pain increases, may call out, moan or groan loudly, or cry.
- Facial expression: May appear sad or frightened, may frown or grimace, especially with activity.
- Body language: May be tense, fidgeting, or pacing, and as pain increases rigid, clenched fists, lying in fetal position, and/or increasingly combative.
- Consolability: Less distractible or consolable.

72. C: Urostomy appliances are usually emptied 4 to 6 times daily, when the pouch is about one-third to one-half full. Allowing the appliance to fill more increases the risk of leakage. Urine should flow continually, but patients can usually establish a routine schedule of emptying the appliance if they maintain a fairly regular schedule of meals and fluid intake. Any change in the usual pattern of urinary output may indicate complications, such as a urinary tract infection or inadequate fluid intake.

73. B: The 3 most common problems associated with takedown of a loop ileostomy are small bowel obstruction, wound infection, and abdominal sepsis. Small bowel obstruction may occur because of twisting of the small intestine or (more commonly) the development of adhesions. The obstruction is usually treated conservatively but may require surgical intervention. The chance of wound infection correlates with wound size, but antibiotic prophylaxis may help prevent. Abdominal sepsis results from anastomotic leak. Localized abscesses may be drained percutaneously but more extensive infection may require laparotomy.

74. B: While good hygiene (washing and drying the anal area after each fecal evacuation) is very important, patients may still develop anal irritation because digestive acids and enzymes are present in the stool because of removal of the colon. If the patient evacuates 8 or more times daily, this increases skin contact with the acids and enzymes and poses a high risk for skin irritation. Patients should be advised to apply skin barrier cream or wipe routinely to protect the skin. Some people complain of itching, which may be relieved with hemorrhoid preparations or aloe vera gel.

75. C: Malabsorption of bile salts may result in increased bowel frequency because they liquefy feces. Bile salts are generally absorbed through the ileum, so malabsorption may occur with resection of the ileum or disease affecting the ileum, such as Crohn's disease. Treatment is usually bile acid sequestrants. For the first 3 months after IPAA, there is minimal intestinal absorptive adaptation, so it may be up to a year before the consistency of the stools is optimal.

76. D: A patient with an ileostomy should be advised to drink about 2000 mL (8 to 10 glasses) of fluid daily because the high output of semi-liquid stool from the colostomy increases the risk of dehydration. Electrolyte levels should be monitored closely and electrolytes replaced as needed. Patients may need to further increase intake when stool output increases. In some cases, patients may be advised to take loperamide to decrease stool output if it remains excessive.

77. C: It is common for residual urine to remain in the bladder after a patient with an orthotopic neobladder urinates; over time, this problem may increase until the neobladder begins to become distended. Therefore, patients should routinely do a clean intermittent catheterization at least one time each month after urinating to check residual volume. About half the women with a neobladder may experience some urinary retention requiring regular or periodic catheterization.

78. C: The ideal protrusion of an ileostomy stoma is about 2 cm (0.8 inches) because this allows for easy fitting and seal of an appliance. A stoma that is flush with the skin is difficult to fit with an appliance and is more likely to leak. If the stoma is too long, it may develop mechanical trauma from the appliance. Stomas are classified as flush (even with or slightly below the skin), moderately protruding (1 to 3 cm), or long (more than 3 cm).

79. B: Sometimes after removal of the colon and rectum, patients experience symptoms of a phantom rectum, similar to the phantom limb experience of amputees. Patients sense rectal pressure and the need to defecate. Often the best solution is for patients to sit on the toilet and bear down as though defecating. These sensations are often most acute in the early months after surgery and usually subside with time. Relaxation exercises and biofeedback may provide relief to some patients.

80. C: A dietary obstruction in a patient with an IPAA usually resolves if the patient stops eating solid foods and drinks only liquids for 24 hours. Massaging the abdomen, taking a hot bath, and walking may help to relieve a blockage. If the blockage persists and the patient develops other symptoms or begins vomiting, then the patient should get medical help. A diet too high in fiber, such as one with many raw fruits or vegetables, may increase the risk of blockage. Fruits and vegetables should be peeled and cooked.

Practice Test #2

Wound Care Practice Questions

1. To reduce the risk of ulcerations, a patient with controlled bilateral peripheral pitting edema and brownish discoloration of skin around the ankles and anterior tibial areas should be advised to

a. stop smoking.
b. wear compression stockings.
c. use off-loading methods.
d. avoid elevating feet above the heart.

2. TransCyte is indicated for treatment of

a. venous ulcers.
b. arterial ulcers.
c. surgical wounds.
d. burns (partial to full thickness).

3. The dietary requirement of protein to promote wound healing is

a. 0.25 to 0.4 g/kg per day.
b. 0.5 to 0.75 g/kg per day.
c. 0.76 to 1.24 g/kg per day.
d. 1.25 to 1.5 g/kg per day.

4. Which infection control precaution(s) should be used when caring for a patient with osteomyelitis and a fistula infected with *Staphylococcus aureus*?

a. standard and contact
b. contact only
c. standard only
d. standard and droplet

5. An example of a wound that will probably undergo secondary healing is

a. a split-thickness graft.
b. an infected wound.
c. an extensive, contaminated dog bite wound.
d. a clean laceration.

6. When considering orthotics and shoe inserts for a patient with a neuropathic foot, which type of insert provides pressure relief?

a. soft
b. semi-soft
c. rigid
d. semi-rigid

7. What does it indicate if a patient with cognitive impairment who is receiving pain medication around the clock has short periods of hyperventilation, cries out frequently, is lying rigidly with fists clenched, and is increasingly combative?

a. inadequate pain control
b. excess sedation from pain medication
c. adverse effects of pain medication
d. increasing dementia

8. The preferred type of exercise to treat scars is

a. strengthening.
b. active-assisted.
c. passive.
d. active.

9. The *BEST* positioning to prevent pressure injuries is

a. 30-degree tilt position, turning every 2 hours.
b. 90-degree lateral side-lying position, turning every 2 hours.
c. prone position on alternating pressure mattress
d. supine position on alternating pressure mattress.

10. Which of the following is *MOST* important during maggot debridement therapy for debridement of an infected pressure injury?

a. maggots must be covered with an occlusive dressing
b. maggots must be left in the wound for 4 hours
c. maggots should be cleaned from the wound with hydrogen peroxide
d. maggots must have an oxygen supply

11. Which is the *BEST* choice of barrier protection for intact skin to protect it from adhesive stripping and small amounts of exudate?

a. skin sealant
b. moister barrier ointment
c. moisture barrier paste
d. solid skin barrier

12. Chemical cauterization with silver nitrate is most commonly used on wounds to

a. debride ulcers.
b. control bleeding.
c. treat hypergranulation.
d. decrease exudate.

13. In describing a wound, the term *slough* refers to

a. softening and irritation caused by skin contact with liquid.
b. Bright pink or red granular-appearing new tissue formed from capillary beds
c. formation of healed tissue from epidermal cells over granulation.
d. soft viscous yellow layer of necrotic tissue that covers and adheres to the wound.

14. When using eutectic mixture of local anesthetics (EMLA) cream to relieve pain during dressing changes, what is the minimum duration of time the cream should be applied before beginning the dressing change?

a. 10 minutes
b. 20 minutes
c. 30 minutes
d. 40 minutes

15. A patient with diabetic ulcers and hemoglobin A1c (HbA1c) of 9.2% with an estimated average glucose (eAG) of 217 should be advised to maintain diabetic control to keep the HbA1c at

a. < 5%.
b. < 6%.
c. < 7%.
d. < 8%.

16. What physical consequences for a leg wound can result from pain?

a. pain may increase peripheral vasoconstriction, decreasing perfusion
b. pain may increase peripheral vasodilation, increasing edema
c. pain may result in increased leukocyte activity
d. pain does not affect wound healing

17. Venous ulcers are commonly

a. deep and circular.
b. superficial and irregular-shaped.
c. necrotic.
d. found on the toes and toe webs.

18. The *BEST* action for a patient who is nearing death and has started to develop a pressure area on the sacral area but moans loudly and is resistive when the nurse assistant tries to turn him is to

a. turn the patient frequently to prevent further skin deterioration.
b. allow the patient to lie undisturbed as much as possible.
c. ask the nurse to increase pain medication so that the patient can be turned.
d. ask to transfer the patient to a bed with an alternating pressure mattress.

19. What preparation is necessary for a patient who has a chronic leg ulcer covered with black eschar and is to have enzymatic debridement with collagenase?

a. thoroughly drying the eschar and surrounding skin
b. applying topical antibiotic
c. scrubbing the wound with hexachlorophene
d. crosshatching the upper layers of the eschar

20. Which of the following should the nurse initially suspect if a wound has remained in the inflammation phase of healing for 10 days without progression and the surrounding skin has remained erythematous and edematous?

a. infection
b. inadequate protein intake
c. secondary trauma
d. immunosuppression

21. The type of wound likely to have the slowest rate of contraction is

a. linear.
b. square.
c. circular.
d. rectangular.

22. Which diagnostic testing is *MOST* indicated for a patient who is a vegan and avoids all gluten-containing foods and legumes as well?

a. prealbumin
b. BUN
c. zinc level
d. vitamin D level

23. Which of the following should be avoided when carrying out measures to prevent friction that may result in pressure injuries?

a. talcum powder
b. skin sealants
c. cornstarch
d. alcohol-based skin barrier

24. When evaluating a patient's nutritional status, what is the number of daily calories usually required for adequate wound healing?

a. 1,000 to 1,200 calories/day
b. 1,500 to 3,500 calories/day
c. 2,000 to 4,000 calories/day
d. 3,000 to 6,000 calories/day

25. When determining the severity level of a pressure injury using the Bates-Jensen Wound Assessment Tool (BWAT), a score of 48 indicates

a. minimal severity.
b. mild severity.
c. moderate severity.
d. critical severity.

26. How would a wound be classified that healed as anticipated for the first week but then appeared to plateau and remained unchanged for the second and third weeks?

a. chronic wound
b. recalcitrant wound
c. stunned wound
d. acute wound

27. Which of the following treatments is initially indicated to relieve weepy, red, itchy atopic dermatitis?

a. topical antihistamine
b. wet aluminum acetate compresses
c. hypoallergenic creams
d. topical antibiotic

28. Which of the following complications may occur if a patient is placed in the prone position to relieve pressure on the hips and spine with the head positioned laterally?

a. injury to the peroneal nerve as well as dislocation of the hip and stress on the lower back and pelvis
b. increased intracranial pressure and increased intraocular pressure
c. diaphragm displaced anteriorly by abdominal viscera resulting in decreased functional residual capacity, especially in elderly patients
d. decreased cerebral circulation and ocular damage

29. The most common site for venous ulcers is

a. medial malleolus.
b. lateral malleolus.
c. great toe.
d. medial aspect of knees.

30. The primary reason for ambulating with an Unna boot is to

a. provide static support to the calf muscle pump.
b. apply dynamic support to the calf muscle pump.
c. apply continuous static compression to the lower leg.
d. apply continuous dynamic support to the lower leg.

31. Which is the *BEST* support surface for a palliative care patient who cannot assume a variety of different positions without experiencing pain and exerting pressure on two existing pressure injuries, stages I and II?

a. static flotation (water)
b. foam
c. alternating air mattress
d. high air loss (air fluidized)

32. Which is the BEST dressing choice to absorb and contain the malodorous drainage from tumor necrosis resulting in a deep ulcerated area with a large amount of exudate?

a. gauze
b. open to air
c. charcoal dressings
d. foam

33. Which fistula management technique is *BEST* to prevent wound contamination from drainage for a large open post-surgical abdominal wound that has developed a fistula in the posterior aspect?

a. simple pouching
b. bridging
c. saddlebagging
d. troughing

34. The SAD (size, area, depth) grading classification is primarily used for

a. neuropathic ulcers.
b. pressure injuries.
c. venous ulcers.
d. arterial ulcers.

35. Which of the following dressings provides moisture to dry wound beds, promotes autolysis of yellow slough, and softens black eschar?

a. hydrocolloids
b. alginate dressings
c. transparent films
d. hydrogels

36. The *BEST* method to assess the degree of undermining is

a. visual inspection.
b. ultrasound.
c. palpation.
d. insert sterile swab.

37. Which of the following lab values is indicative of dehydration?

a. BUN/creatinine ratio: 28:1
b. urine specific gravity 1.001
c. BUN: 7 mg/dL
d. serum osmolality 290 mOsm/kg

38. At which stage in the healing of an incisional wound should a healing ridge be evident?

a. inflammatory days 1 to 4
b. proliferative days 5 to 9
c. proliferative days 10 to 14
d. proliferative to remodeling day 15 onward

39. When staging tissue damage from irradiation, how would moist, blistering tissue with epidermal tissue loss, serous drainage, and increased pain because of nerve exposure be classified?

a. stage I
b. stage II
c. stage III
d. stage IV

40. What is the *BEST* debridement choice for a pressure injury with hard, dry, black adherent eschar covering 75% of the wound?

a. autolytic with transparent film dressing
b. autolytic with hydrocolloid or hydrogel
c. sharp
d. enzymatic

41. Which class of compression stockings (such as Jobst or Therapress Duo) is indicated after edema is controlled to prevent venous ulcers for those at risk?

a. class 1: 20 to 30 mm Hg
b. class 2: 30 to 40 mm Hg
c. class 3: 40 to 50 mm Hg
d. class 4: 50 to 60 mm Hg

42. After treatment is discontinued, when will myopia resolve if it developed as a complication of hyperbaric oxygen therapy?

a. never
b. within 1 to 2 years
c. within 6 months
d. within 6 weeks

43. What is the *BEST* solution for applying negative-pressure wound therapy (NPWT) to a large sacral wound that extends between the gluteal folds, preventing the adhesive dressing from sealing and resulting in a leak?

a. cut foam large enough to fill the area where the leak occurs
b. discontinue NPWT and institute a different kind of therapy
c. apply skin prep to the skin before applying adhesive
d. apply stoma paste to facilitate a seal

44. When doing a pressure wound assessment using the Sussman Wound Healing Tool (SWHT), which of the following would be considered attributes that are "not good" for healing?

a. fibroplasia
b. contraction
c. adherence
d. erythema

45. Patient goals are developed from

a. the problem list.
b. physician orders.
c. the patient interview.
d. standardized goals associated with diagnosis.

46. As circulation decreases in the lower extremities, what hair distribution changes occur?

a. none
b. hair is lost on toes only
c. hair is lost proximally
d. hair is lost distally

47. Infrared thermography is especially useful for evaluating

a. extent of pressure injuries.
b. extent of infection.
c. risk of neuropathic ulcers.
d. phase of wound healing.

48. Which of the following is generally the best method of realigning a 3 cm skin tear (Payne-Martin category I, flap type) on the forearm on an 80-year-old patient?

a. tissue glue
b. sutures
c. staples
d. pressure dressing

49. During the monofilament test on the dorsum of the foot, the inability to perceive which force level is considered the threshold for loss of protective sensation?

a. 3.61
b. 4.17
c. 5.07
d. 6.1

50. What precaution is necessary when using pulsatile lavage with suction (PLWS) for mechanical debridement?

a. allow only close family members in room
b. use only if the patient's bed can be curtained off from others
c. disinfect room prior to treatment
d. use only in a private room

51. When conducting a pulse exam of the lower extremities, a pulse that is felt but diminished would be graded as

a. 1+.
b. 2+.
c. 3+.
d. 4+.

52. At what angle should the Doppler probe be placed over the artery when assessing the brachial or ankle systolic pressure for the Ankle Brachial Index (ABI)?

a. 10 degrees
b. 30 degrees
c. 45 degrees
d. 90 degrees

53. The optimal sitting position is

a. 95 degrees at hip and knee and 90 to 95 degrees at ankles.
b. 90 degrees at hip, knees, and ankles.
c. 90 degrees at hip, 95 degrees at knees and ankles.
d. 90 degrees at hip and knees and 95 degrees at ankles.

54. Sharp debridement would be recommended for which of the following?

a. large pressure injury covered with moist necrotic tissue with evidence of increasing cellulitis
b. large ischemic ulcer on ankle with evidence of cellulitis
c. stable pressure area on heel covered by black eschar
d. small pressure injury on right hip covered with yellow slough

55. Which type of wound usually produces the most exudate?

a. arterial ulcer
b. diabetic/neuropathic ulcer
c. pressure injury
d. venous ulcer

56. Which is the *BEST* debridement choice for a pressure injury with soft, stringy, adherent yellow slough covering 33% of the wound bed?

a. enzymatic
b. sharp
c. autolytic with hydrocolloids or hydrogels
d. autolytic with transparent film dressing

57. Apligraf, a biological skin substitute, is indicated for which of the following?

a. first-line treatment for infected venous ulcer
b. diabetic ulcer (2-month duration) with muscle, tendon, capsule, or bone exposure
c. diabetic ulcer (1-month duration) with no muscle, tendon, capsule, or bone exposure
d. refractory venous leg ulcer (2-week duration)

58. For which of the following wounds would the use of a topical antiseptic be contraindicated?

a. chronic venous ulcer
b. second- and third-degree burns
c. dog bite injury
d. traumatic wound contaminated with debris

59. What is usually the appropriate pH to maintain in a wound and periwound tissue?

a. 4 to 5
b. 5 to 6
c. 6 to 7
d. 7 to 8

60. When using becaplermin gel to treat a diabetic ulcer, the gel should be left on the wound each day for

a. 2 hours.
b. 8 hours.
c. 12 hours.
d. 24 hours.

61. What is the most likely treatment for a patient with venous insufficiency who develops pain and tenderness along the saphenous vein in the lower leg but without erythema or swelling?

a. compression and NSAIDs
b. warfarin or low-molecular-weight heparin
c. bedrest and oral antibiotics
d. compression and bedrest

62. Platelet-derived wound healing factor (PDWHF), such as AutoloGel, is derived from

a. pooled donor platelets.
b. single unrelated-donor platelets.
c. single related donor platelets
d. patient's own platelets.

63. The correct procedure for obtaining a wound drainage specimen for aerobic culture is to

a. aspirate the wound drainage with a syringe without a needle.
b. aspirate the wound drainage with a syringe with a needle.
c. rotate a sterile swab in the drainage site.
d. wipe the wound from side to side with a sterile swab.

64. Which of the following topical medications is effective against bacteria, viruses, and fungi?

a. cadexomer iodine
b. nystatin
c. silver sulfadiazine
d. metronidazole

65. Which of the following medications may contribute to bilateral peripheral edema?

a. calcium channel blockers
b. loop diuretics
c. tricyclic antidepressants
d. acetaminophen

66. What should be done prior to sharp debridement for a wound covered with dry eschar?

a. no further prep necessary
b. mechanical debridement
c. autolytic or enzymatic debridement
d. pulsed lavage with suction

67. What is the most likely cause of a diabetic patient experiencing pain and diffuse swelling in the right foot, especially over the tarsometatarsal joint, with increased skin temperature of 5°F?

a. ischemia
b. deep compartmental infection
c. gout
d. Charcot arthropathy

68. An effective alternative to pressure dressing to treat hypertrophic scarring in a small area to which pressure cannot be easily applied is

a. massage.
b. silicone polymer gel.
c. tissue expanders.
d. surgical excision.

69. The Vancouver Scar Scale to Measure Scar Formation assesses pigmentation and vascularity as well as

a. location and height.
b. location and deformity.
c. thickness and surface.
d. pliability and height.

70. After acute surgery, the remodeling phase of wound healing of the incision usually lasts

a. 2 to 4 months.
b. 6 to 12 months.
c. 1 to 2 years.
d. 2 to 4 years.

71. What is the National Pressure Injury Advisory Panel (NPIAP) stage of a pressure injury that exhibits nonblanchable erythema and decreased skin temperature but intact skin?

a. stage I
b. stage II
c. stage III
d. stage IV

72. The best solution for a patient who has a small coccygeal pressure injury and can turn from side to side but bottoms out on her foam support surface and tends to slide down in bed is

a. static air flotation device.
b. static water flotation device.
c. dynamic alternating air device.
d. low-air-loss device.

73. For maintenance of skin to prevent drying and cracking, the choice that provides the longest duration of moisturizing is

a. lotions.
b. ointments.
c. creams.
d. oil bath.

74. Atrophie blanche lesions are indicative of

a. venous insufficiency.
b. arterial insufficiency.
c. lipodermatosclerosis.
d. lymphedema.

75. The best intervention for a diabetic patient with hammertoe and neuropathy to prevent ulceration is

a. tube foam.
b. sandal use instead of closed-toe shoes.
c. metatarsal pads.
d. crepe sole shoes.

76. With the Sussman Wound Healing Protocol for high voltage pulsed current (HVPC) treatment, the duration and frequency of treatment for inflammation are

a. 60 minutes 5 to 7 times weekly for 1 week and then 3 times weekly for 1 week.
b. 60 minutes 5 to 7 times weekly.
c. 60 minutes 3 to 5 times weekly.
d. 60 minutes 3 times weekly.

77. Which of the following can be used to stimulate erythema and restart the epithelialization phase of healing?

a. vitamin C
b. infrared radiation
c. laser
d. ultraviolet C light

78. What organism should be suspected if a burn wound develops increased thick greenish exudate with a foul, musty, fruity odor?

a. *Clostridioides difficile*
b. *Staphylococcus aureus*
c. *Streptococcus pyogenes*
d. *Pseudomonas aeruginosa*

79. What does it mean if a patient complains of increased pain during a pulsed short-wave diathermy treatment?

a. inadequate heating
b. unrelated to therapy
c. expected response
d. excessive heating

80. When evaluating edema, pitting to 4 mm that persists for 10 to 15 seconds would be classified on a 1- to 4-point scale as

a. 1+.
b. 2+.
c. 3+.
d. 4+.

Wound Care Answers and Explanations

1. B: Therapeutic compression stockings (class II, 30 to 40 mm Hg) are used to prevent ulceration in those with varicose veins and stable venous insufficiency (indicated by brownish discoloration) after edema is controlled or with existing ulcers when edema recedes. Patients should also elevate feet when sitting. Therapy may include lying down and elevating the affected limb above the heart for 1 to 2 hours two times daily and during the night. While everyone should stop smoking, it is more critical for those with peripheral arterial insufficiency.

2. D: TransCyte, which uses human neonatal fibroblasts on a nylon mesh protected by a silicone layer, is indicated for partial- or full-thickness burns as a temporary covering before autografting as well as for partial-thickness burns that will not require autografting. TransCyte must be applied to a clean wound base that has been freshly debrided. After application, TransCyte is secured with compression dressing or negative pressure and can last up to 100 days, although it must be removed if infection occurs or fluid begins to accumulate below the TransCyte.

3. D: Protein is critical for wound healing, and because metabolic rate increases in response to a wound, protein needs to increase. Diet requirements for wound healing are 1.25 to 1.5 g/kg per day. A patient weighing 150 lb/68 kg would usually require about 60 g of protein daily but that need would increase to 85 to 102 g daily, so the patient would need to markedly increase intake of high-protein foods or take dietary supplements. Meat, for example, contains only 7 g of protein per ounce.

4. A: Standard precautions, such as washing hands and wearing gloves and personal protective equipment (PPE) as needed for contact with bodily fluids, are used with all patients. However, patients with draining wounds, such as a fistula, should also have contact precautions, which require the use of PPE, including gown and gloves for all contact with the patient or the patient's immediate environment. The patient should be maintained in a private room or cohorted and should remain more than 3 feet away from other patients.

5. B: Secondary healing: Leaving the wound open to close through granulation and epithelialization. Used with contaminated, "dirty," or infected wounds to prevent abscess formation and allow drainage. Primary healing: Involves a wound that is surgically closed by suturing, flaps, or split or full-thickness grafts to completely cover the wound. Used for surgeries or repair of wounds or lacerations, especially when the wound is essentially "clean." Tertiary healing: Involves first debriding the wound and allowing it to begin healing while open and then later closing the wound. Used for contaminated wounds, such as severe animal bites, or wounds related to mixed trauma.

6. D: Semi-rigid inserts provide some cushioning as well as pressure relief. Soft inserts are used primarily for cushioning and to absorb shock. Rigid inserts, usually made from plastic, are used to maintain alignment or control abnormal motion. Accommodative inserts are inserts of multiple layers, reduced by half with compression. Shoes should be made of soft leather and should have enough depth to allow for inserts. Other modifications can include rocker soles, heel wrap, lateral flare, and mid-foot bolsters.

7. A: The patient is exhibiting nonverbal indications of pain. The Pain Assessment in Advanced Dementia (PAINAD) scale is as follows:

- Respirations: Rapid and labored breathing as pain increases, with short periods of hyperventilation or Cheyne-Stokes respirations.
- Vocalization: Negative in speech or speaking quietly and reluctantly, may moan or groan. As pain increases, may call out, moan or groan loudly, or cry.

- Facial expression: May appear sad or frightened, may frown or grimace, especially with activity.
- Body language: May be tense, fidgeting, or pacing, and as pain increases rigid, clenched fists, or lying in fetal position and increasingly combative.
- Consolability: Less distractible or consolable.

8. D: Active exercise is the preferred type to treat scars because the patient remains in control of the exercise regimen and the degree of stretching, although the exercise program should be prescribed for the patient and monitored for effectiveness. With active assist, the therapist or equipment (such as weights and pulleys) assists the patient to complete an exercise, but the patient should be as active as possible. With passive exercise, the patient remains dependent on others to carry out the stretching exercises. Strengthening exercises are indicated if muscle strength is impaired.

9. A: Because the 90-degree side-lying lateral position results in ischemia over bony prominences, patients should be positioned in the 30-degree tilt position because this causes less circulatory impairment. Goals for repositioning and a turning schedule of at least every 2 hours should be established for each individual, with documentation required. Devices, such as pillows or foam, should be used to correctly position patients so that bony prominences are protected and not in direct contact with each other. Pressure can occur even with alternating pressure mattresses.

10. D: Because maggots are living things, they must have an oxygen supply, so they cannot be covered with hydrogels or other occlusive dressings. Maggots are applied to an open wound, but should not be applied to exposed vessels because they may cause bleeding. A special cage is applied to encase the maggots and allow air to circulate. The maggots are left in place for 48 hours and then wiped out with gauze, and then the wound is irrigated with NS.

11. A: Skin sealants are film-forming barriers composed of a polymer in a fast-drying solvent, applied every 1 to 4 days, depending on the product. When the sealant is applied to the skin, the solvent (often isopropyl alcohol) dissolves, leaving the transparent plasticized polymer barrier over the tissue. It may be applied to intact or irritated tissue, although there may be some discomfort from the alcohol solvent contact with broken skin. Sealants can be used to protect skin from exudate, urine, stool, chemicals, and adhesive stripping. Sealants are applied with wipes, wands, or sprays.

12. C: Chemical cauterization with silver nitrate is sometimes used to treat hypergranulation. Cauterization uses heat to burn or sear abnormal cells in order to destroy them. Silver nitrate sticks are wet with water to activate and are then gently rolled for a short time over the tissue to be treated. The most common use for chemical cauterization in wounds or skin lesions is to control hypergranulation tissue that grows in wounds, especially about stomas. Hypergranulation tissue is often friable and bleeds easily. Treatment may be repeated 2 times daily for 1 to 4 days until excess tissue sloughs.

13. D: Slough: Soft viscous yellow layer of necrotic tissue that covers and adheres to the wound. Granulation: Bright pink or red granular appearing new tissue formed from capillary beds. Eschar: Dark brown or black leathery necrotic tissue. Epithelization: Formation of healed tissue from epidermal cells over granulation. Maceration: Softening and irritation caused by contact with liquid. Eschar: Dark brown or black leathery necrotic tissue. Necrosis: Dead tissue. Cellulitis: Inflammation of tissue, usually with edema and pronounced erythema.

14. C: EMLA cream provides good pain control. The wound is first cleansed and then the cream is applied thickly (1/4 inch), extending about 1/2 inch past the wound to the periwound tissue. The wound is then covered with plastic wrap, which is secured and left in place for about 30 minutes. The wrapped time may be extended to 45 to 60 minutes if necessary to completely numb the tissue. The tissue should remain numb for about 1 hour after the plastic wrap is removed, allowing time for the wound to be cleansed, debrided, and/or redressed.

15. C: Generally, diabetic patients are advised to maintain an HbA1c < 7% (154 eAG). Nondiabetic patients usually range from 4% to 5.6% with levels > 5.7% to 6.4% indicating prediabetes, and 6.5% or higher indicating diabetes. When glucose levels are elevated, glucose attaches to hemoglobin molecules on red blood cells, which survive an average of 120 days. The longer glucose levels are elevated, the more glucose attaches, so if elevation is prolonged, it will be reflected in the glucose levels of hemoglobin. Thus, testing for HbA1c provides an evaluation of average serum glucose levels over a 2- to 3-month period.

16. A: Pain can result in peripheral vasoconstriction, decreasing perfusion of tissue and impairing leukocyte activity. This, in turn, depresses angiogenesis, further impairing healing of the wound and continuing the cycle of pain. Pain assessment should be done regularly, allowing the patient to describe the type and extent of pain, as well as response to analgesia. Poor perfusion and infection increase pain, so measures should aim at increasing circulation/oxygenation of the wound and assessing for signs of infection. Increasing fluid intake and providing proper nutrition improve wound condition and reduce pain. Pain medications should be given as needed and prior to dressing changes.

17. B: Venous ulcers are typically superficial irregular ulcers on the medial or lateral malleolus and sometimes the anterior tibial area, causing varying degrees of pain. Surrounding skin often has brownish discoloration. Edema is moderate to severe. Arterial ulcers are painful, deep, circular, often necrotic ulcers found on toe tips, toe webs, heels or other pressure areas. There is often rubor on dependency but pallor on foot elevation, and skin is pale, shiny, and cool. Edema is minimal.

18. B: When a patient is nearing death, the most important consideration is comfort, even if this means that some routine patient care, such as turning the patient, must be set aside. The patient should be allowed to lie undisturbed as much as possible. Pain medication is usually decreased as a patient nears death; increasing the medication may result in increased adverse effects. The process of transferring a patient to another bed may cause discomfort and distress.

19. D: Chemical debridement with enzymes is used for chronic wounds (burns, ulcers) with necrotic tissue and eschar. However, the enzymes (collagenase and papain/urea) require a moist environment, so the eschar must be crosshatched through the upper layers before the enzyme is administered. The pH must remain between 6 and 8 or the enzyme action is inactivated. Other causes of inactivation include hexachlorophene, Burrow's solution, and heavy metal ions. Collagenase is applied once daily, either directly to the wound for deep wounds or to gauze packing for shallow wounds.

20. A: When a wound remains in the inflammation phase of healing and does not progress to the proliferation phase, the most common reason is infection of the tissue. Inflammation may also be prolonged when necrotic tissue is present. The wound should be evaluated with culture and sensitivities to determine what interventions may be needed. Depending on the size of the wound and the degree of infection, an infected wound may be treated with IV, oral, or topical antibiotics.

21. C: Wound contraction occurs during phase III of healing. Proliferation, when a ring of myofibroblasts develops beneath the skin, contracts the tissue. Circular wounds tend to contract slowly, while linear wounds (such as a surgical incision) contract rapidly, with square and rectangular wounds contracting at an intermediate rate. If contraction occurs too rapidly, it can result in excessive scarring, so contraction should be monitored and controlled, especially in areas such as the face, to avoid disfigurement, and hands, to avoid loss of mobility.

22. C: Because the patient's diet excludes animal protein as well as gluten-containing foods (such as wheat products) and legumes, the patient is at risk for zinc deficiency and should have zinc levels assessed. Supplementation should be provided, usually 110 to 220 mg of zinc gluconate or zinc sulfate 3 times daily. Zinc deficiency often coincides with vitamins A and D deficiency as well, so supplementation with these vitamins may be considered as well. Because the patient's diet is so restrictive, the patient should be evaluated for anorexia, which can also be an indication of zinc deficiency.

23. A: Friction by itself results only in damage to the epidermis and dermis, such as abrasions or denudement referred to as "sheet burn." Friction and pressure can combine, however, to form pressure injuris, so preventive measures are critical. Talcum powder may result in skin abrasion, so it should be avoided, although cornstarch can be applied to the skin or bed linens. Skin sealants and alcohol-based or non–alcohol-based skin barriers as well as skin lubricants may also provide protection from friction.

24. B: Adequate wound healing usually requires an intake of 1,500 to 3,500 calories per day, depending on the patient's age, size, and general condition. A lower caloric intake may restrict the protein necessary to promote the development of collagen and wound healing. If carbohydrate intake is too low, then the body may utilize protein for energy. Fats are necessary for construction of the cell membrane, and deficiency impairs healing. Patients need a well-balanced diet with vitamins and minerals. Vitamin C, vitamin A, iron, and copper are all important in the development of collagen.

25. D: A BWAT score of 42 indicates critical severity. BWAT comprises 11 categories: size, depth, edges, undermining, necrotic tissue type, necrotic tissue amount, exudate type, exudate amount, periwound skin color, peripheral tissue edema, peripheral tissue induration, granulation tissue, and epithelialization. Each category is scored from 1 to 5 with lower scores indicating lower severity. Scores are totaled to indicate severity:

- 13 to 20: Minimal.
- 21 to 30: Mild.
- 31 to 40: Moderate.
- 41 to 65: Critical.

26. C: Stunned wound: Appears to be healing well initially but then reaches a plateau and does not progress past that point of healing. Acute wound: From surgery or trauma and usually heals within an expected period of time without complications. Chronic wound: Persists more than 30 days and fails to progress. Some may never heal. Recalcitrant wound: Fails to follow a normal progression of healing and is difficult to manage because it fails to heal even with various treatments.

27. B: Wet aluminum acetate compresses are used to treat weepy lesions associated with atopic dermatitis. Atopic dermatitis (eczema) is a chronic inflammatory superficial skin disorder. It is related to allergies and associated with xerosis, which is dry skin with impaired barrier function. It is associated with dry or cold weather, central heating (which dries the air), and irritation caused by soaps and other skin cleaners. Skin is often red and itchy, and vesicles may develop, ooze, and crust. Skin may be rough, cracked, and scaly. Over time, skin may darken and thicken, and lichenification (markings from chronic scratching) may develop.

28. D: In the prone position, blood may pool in the extremities, and pressure on the abdomen may result in a decrease in BP, preload, and cardiac output. Respiratory effort increases, and lung compliance decreases. The head may be turned laterally, or if contraindicated because of arthritis or cerebrovascular disease, maintained in neutral position. Head positioned sharply to one side or the other may interfere with cerebral circulation. If head is turned laterally, then the dependent eye must be observed carefully for external compression that may cause ocular damage.

29. A: The medial malleolus is the most common site for venous ulcers because it is the distal point along the hydrostatic column of pressure and is distal to the calf pump and near the distal end of the lesser saphenous vein. Because of these factors, the medial malleolus is the point where venous pressure is the highest. However, ulcers may occur at any point between the knees and the ankle, so controlling edema and reducing venous hypertension is necessary as preventive measures.

30. A: The Unna boot is not in itself a compression device because the wrapping is applied firmly but with little tension. The patient must ambulate in order to gain benefit from the Unna boot, which becomes quite rigid after it is wrapped with elastic and provides static support. Because of the rigidity, the boot forces the pressure from muscle contractions inward as the person ambulates, and this pressure causes the one-way bicuspid valves of the calf muscle pump to open, forcing the blood upward and out of the area, reducing edema.

31. C: The alternating air mattress is a dynamic support surface and especially useful for palliative care patients who cannot be moved easily without pain because it may assist with tissue perfusion even when patients are immobile. The support surface should be assessed with the patient in various positions for bottoming out by placing a flat hand beneath the patient's pressure points and ensuring there is at least an inch of support. Alternating air mattresses may result in moisture retention and heat accumulation.

32. C: While there are multiple ways to manage wounds with heavy exudate, in the context of malodorous wounds from tumor necrosis, charcoal dressings are most effective in both managing the exudate and absorbing the odor which can provide immense emotional relief to patients.

33. B: Bridging is a method to contain fistula drainage while protecting the wound from the exudate. A bridge is built with small pieces of barrier wafers, layering them until they are equal to the depth of the wound. This bridge is then adhered to the wound with barrier paste and an ostomy pouch is then cut to fit the opening of the fistula. The ostomy pouch is applied to the intact skin on one side and the bridge on the other.

34. A: The SAD (size, area, depth) grading classification system, a modification of Wagner, is used for neuropathic ulcers. It includes evidence of sepsis, arteriopathy, and denervation as well. Ulcers are graded from grade 0 (no evidence of pathology). Grade 1 ulcers are < 10 mm^2 and extend into subcutaneous tissue. Exudate or superficial slough is present, and pulses are absent or diminished. Sensation is reduced. Grade 2 ulcers are 10 to 20 mm^2 and can involve the tendons, joints, or periosteum. Cellulitis is present, but pulses may be absent. Grade 3 ulcers are > 30 mm^2 and involve bones and joints. Osteomyelitis, Charcot foot, and gangrene are evident.

35. D: Hydrogels are moisture-retentive, so they provide moisture to dry wound beds and promote autolysis of yellow slough and softening of black eschar. They are effective for partial- or full-thickness wounds with small amounts of exudate but are contraindicated with large amounts of exudate. They can be used with infected wounds. They increase risk of yeast infections and may contribute to periwound maceration. Hydrogels are applied directly to the wound and covered with secondary dressings.

36. D: The best method to assess the degree of undermining is to insert a sterile swab into the undermined area, note the depth on the swab, and then measure it. Undermined areas may remain intact even though the tissue is damaged. In that case, the tissue should be palpated as it may feel spongy with the degree of undermining estimated. Undermining should be reported according to its relation to the open wound by reference to a clock face: "Undermining of 2.5 cm width extends from 1 o'clock to 2 o'clock."

37. A: BUN/creatinine ratio: > 25:1 indicates dehydration and < 10:1 overhydration.

Urine specific gravity: > 1.028 g/mL indicates dehydration and < 1.002 g/mL overhydration.

BUN: > 35 mg/dL indicates dehydration and < 7 mg/dL overhydration.

Serum osmolality: > 303 mOsm/kg indicates dehydration and > 320 mOsm/kg overhydration.

Serum sodium: > 145 mEq/L indicates dehydration and < 130 mEq/L overhydration.

Normal fluid requirements are 30 mL/kg of body weight or a minimum of 1,500 mL daily, although patients with draining wounds may require extra fluids.

38. B: Collagen deposit should create a palpable healing ridge along the incision during the phase of proliferation (days 5 to 9), and the ridge should be evident along the full length of the incision by day 9. It usually extends to about 1 cm on each side of the wound. If there is no evidence of the healing ridge by day 9, then the wound is at increased risk of dehiscence and infection. Sutures are usually removed from most wounds between days 5 and 9.

39. C: Staging of tissue damage from irradiation:

I	Inflammation results in increased edema and capillary permeability with erythema, itching, burning, and/or pain.
II	Skin is dry, itchy, and scaly, and epidermis begins to slough because of damage to basal epidermal cells and glands.
III	Epidermis continues to slough off, leaving skin moist and blistering with serous drainage and increased pain because nerves are exposed.
IV	Tissue changes include hair loss, atrophy, pigment changes, and ulcerations.

40. A: The best debridement choice for a pressure injury with hard, dry, black adherent eschar covering 75% to 100% of the wound is autolytic with transparent film dressing because the dressing traps fluid without absorbing it, more rapidly hydrating the eschar. The eschar should be crosshatched prior to application of the dressing to facilitate autolysis, and the circulation should be evaluated. Hydrogels and hydrocolloids may also be used; however, because they have absorptive properties, autolysis may take longer to be effective.

41. B: Class 2 compression stocking should be used after edema is controlled. Compression stockings are classified according to the degree of compression:

- Class 1: 20 to 30 mm Hg, used for treatment of varicose veins.
- Class 2: 30 to 40 mm Hg, used to prevent venous ulcers for those at risk.
- Class 3: 40 to 50 mm Hg, used to treat refractory venous ulcers and lymphedema.
- Class 4: 50 to 60 mm Hg, used to treat lymphedema.

42. C: Myopia may occur with hyperbaric oxygen therapy because the pressure in the eye changes the eye shape. This usually resolves with the eye returning to its normal shape within 6 months after treatment is discontinued. People with cataracts may also experience increased clouding of vision. Other complications of hyperbaric oxygen therapy include barotrauma (which may result in ruptured eardrum and organ damage) and oxygen toxicity (which may cause CNS symptoms, such as hallucination and seizures).

43. D: NPWT is often applied to areas where the tissue is discontinuous or skin folds interfere with adherence of the adhesive dressing, so the best solution is to apply stoma paste to the area where the leak is occurring to create a bridge to which to apply the clear adhesive dressing. The foam should be cut to fit the wound so that when negative pressure is applied (tested by pressing down with a finger) the foam does not overlap the wound because this may result in maceration of the tissue.

44. D: SWHT was developed to monitor healing of pressure wounds. Part I assesses 5 tissue attributes classified as "not good" for healing: hemorrhage, maceration, undermining, erythema, and necrosis. It also assesses 5 tissue attributes that are "good" for healing: adherence, granulation, contraction, sustained contraction, and epithelialization. Part II assesses wound depth and tunneling/undermining. Additional attributes include describing the location of the wound and the healing phase as chronic, acute, or absent.

45. A: Goals are developed from the problem list that is generated as part of the plan of care, based on patient interview, history, physical exam, and medical records. Goals should be specifically related to the problem, measurable by some method, and attainable. Goals may focus on three areas:

- Resolution: "Pulse rates will not exceed 90 at rest."
- Preventing deterioration or further complications: "Patient will remain at current weight."
- Palliation/patient comfort: "Patient will not experience breakthrough pain."

46. D: As circulation decreases in the lower extremities, hair distribution is loss distally, so assessing hair distribution is one measure to evaluate impaired circulation. Because hair follicles provide epidermal cells that are important for resurfacing of partial-thickness wounds, the absence of hair can negatively affect healing, especially in areas where hair has been lost. The hair on the great toes should be assessed because lack of hair (if not shaven) indicates circulatory impairment. The hair distribution on the leg should be evaluated to determine the most distal area of hair growth.

47. C: Infrared thermography is especially useful for evaluating the risk of neuropathic ulcers. While fever strips are often used to evaluate increased temperature at a wound site, they are not as sensitive to measure subtle changes. People at risk for neuropathic ulcers often have an impaired immune system, so the usual signs of inflammation (erythema at the site of damaged tissue) may not be evident, but the temperature of the area may be increased and detectable by infrared thermography.

48. A: Because Payne-Martin category I injuries align well, tissue glue is probably the best choice because it minimizes drainage and keeps the flap securely in place. Mature skin is generally more friable than younger skin, so sutures and/or staples may cause more trauma and should be avoided if possible. A pressure dressing alone may not provide adequate alignment because dressings can shift. Also, dressings may adhere to the wound, causing increased trauma during removal. When adhesive strips are used, they must be spaced to allow for drainage.

49. C: The force level considered the threshold for loss of protective sensation with the monofilament test on the dorsum of the foot is 5.07; inability to perceive a force level of 4.56 on the plantar surface of the foot indicates loss of protective sensation. Inability to perceive force level of 3.61 is considered within normal parameters, but those who cannot perceive 5.07 force level are at increased risk because their ability to use protective sensations is limited.

50. D: Because microorganisms can become aerosolized during treatment with PLWS, the patient must be treated in a private room with the door closed to ensure contamination does not spread; curtaining off the patient is not adequate. There should be no visitors or family present during treatment and any other open wounds, ports, IVs, or other tubes on the patient should be covered. The nurse should wear appropriate PPE. The room must be thoroughly disinfected after treatment.

51. A: A pulse that is felt but diminished is graded as 1+. The pulse exam for vascular evaluation of the lower extremities should be conducted bilaterally with the femoral, popliteal, dorsalis, pedis, and posterior tibial artery pulses. The popliteal pulse is most easily assessed with the patient in the prone position. Pulses are graded from 0 to 4+:

- 0: No pulse palpable.
- 1+: Pulse is weak and difficult to palpate.
- 2+: Pulse is normal.
- 3+: Pulse is full.
- 4+: Pulse is abnormally bounding, aneurysmal.

52. C: ABI procedure (do bilaterally and use higher readings):

- Apply blood pressure cuff to one arm, palpate brachial pulse, and place conductivity gel over artery.
- Place tip of a Doppler device at a 45-degree angle into gel at brachial artery, and listen for pulse sound.
- Inflate cuff until pulse sound ceases and then inflate 20 mm Hg above that point.
- Release air and listen for return of pulse sound for brachial systolic pressure.
- Repeat same procedure on each ankle with cuff applied above the malleoli and gel over the posterior tibial pulse for ankle systolic pressure.
- Divide ankle systolic pressure by brachial systolic pressure to obtain the ABI.

53. A: The optimal sitting position is 95 degrees at hip and knees and 90 to 95 degrees at the ankles. The 95-degree angle at the hip and knees allows the patient to sit upright while interfering less with perfusion than when a patient is sitting at 90 degrees. Patients should be carefully evaluated for range of motion and ability to sit in an upright position as modifications must be made for those with limited range of motion. Feet should be supported when patients are in sitting position.

54. A: Sharp debridement would be recommended for the large pressure injury covered with moist necrotic tissue with evidence of cellulitis as it may convert the wound from necrotic to acute and clean, promoting healing. Sharp debridement may be done in conjunction with other methods, such as enzymatic, mechanic, or autolytic debridement, to soften eschar. Ischemic ulcers should not undergo sharp debridement and stable pressure areas covered by black eschar on the heels are usually left intact because the eschar provides some protection. Small pressure injuries with yellow slough may be treated with other forms of debridement.

55. D: Because venous wounds are usually associated with peripheral edema, they tend to produce the most exudate throughout the healing process, so providing gradient compression to reduce edema is an important aspect of treatment. Venous wounds may be covered with yellow fibrinous material that can appear to be exudate. Arterial wounds tend to be dry or to have slight exudate. Neuropathic wounds usually have minimal serous or serosanguineous exudate. Pressure injuries have varying amounts of exudate, depending on the wound characteristics.

56. C: Because slough provides a moist environment, the best choice for debridement is autolytic with hydrocolloids or hydrogels because they have absorptive properties to contain exudate while maintaining the moist environment to facilitate autolysis. Enzymatic debridement may also be considered but the agent chosen must be effective against collagen and protein and the surrounding skin must be protected from the enzyme and exudate, or maceration may occur. In some cases, sharp debridement may be done, often in conjunction with autolytic debridement.

57. C: Apligraf is FDA-approved for diabetic ulcers of more than 2 weeks duration with no muscle, tendon, capsule, or bone exposure, as well as venous leg ulcers that have been refractory to other treatments and persisted for more than a month. Apligraf is composed of two layers. The epidermal layer is from neonatal keratinocytes (from neonatal foreskin), and the dermal layer is from bovine collagen seeded with neonatal fibroblasts. Apligraf should not be used in infected wounds or with necrosis.

58. A: Topical antiseptics are generally contraindicated in the treatment of chronic wounds, such as a venous ulcer, as they have little value and may cause injury to tissue. Topical antiseptics only affect bacteria on the wound surface but cannot reach infected tissue, so wound infection is better treated with systemic antibiotics. Topical antiseptics, however, are used with acute wounds, such as dog bite and other traumatic contaminated wounds, to prevent infection, and may be indicated in patients who are immunocompromised. They are also routinely used with burns because necrotic tissue can lead to infection.

59. B: Wounds and periwound tissue should be maintained with an acid pH of 5 to 6, so most skin cleansers, which tend to be alkaline, should be avoided in favor of irrigating the wound with water or normal saline. Any cleansing materials should be used at body temperature (lukewarm) because cold solutions may interfere with wound perfusion. Direct contact with granulating tissue should be minimal. Skin or wound cleansers with surfactant properties, along with irrigants, may help to remove debris.

60. C: Becaplermin (Regranex Gel) is a growth factor used to promote wound healing of diabetic/neuropathic ulcers that extend into or beyond the subcutaneous tissue but have adequate perfusion. The wound is coated with 1/16 inch of gel and covered with gauze moistened with NS, which is left in place for 12 hours. Then the dressing is removed, and the wound is irrigated with NS and covered with gauze moistened with NS for the next 12 hours. This procedure is repeated daily.

61. A: Pain and tenderness along the saphenous vein in the lower leg are usually associated with superficial phlebitis and treated with compression and NSAIDs and continued ambulation as risk for development of deep vein thrombosis (DVT) is low. However, if erythema, swelling, and marked pain occur, this may indicate DVT, which should be confirmed with Doppler. DVT may be treated with anticoagulation (warfarin, heparin) or thrombolysis, although thrombolysis increases risk of hemorrhage or stroke. The affected leg is elevated with use of a compression device to reduce swelling.

62. D: Platelet-derived wound healing factor (PDWHF), such as AutoloGel, is derived from the patient's own platelets, so it is prepared individually. It is used to initiate coagulation and provide growth factors to improve and hasten healing. The gel is applied topically and left in place for 5 days, after which an alternative dressing is applied for 7 days and then the cycle repeated until wound healing occurs. AutoloGel has been used effectively to treat diabetic neuropathic ulcers involving deep structures, such as tendons and fascia.

63. C: Aerobic cultures are for bacteria that grow when exposed to air, so the appropriate method is to remove a sterile swab from a culture tube, rotate it gently in an area of drainage in the wound, return the swab to the culture tube, crush the ampule containing medium, and push the swab into the medium because this helps to keep the bacteria viable until the sample can be analyzed. Anaerobic cultures are taken from deeper in the wound and aspirated with a syringe without a needle.

64. A: Cadexomer iodine prepared as a paste, powder, or ointment is effective against a broad range of bacteria (MRSA, *S. aureus, Streptococcus, Pseudomonas)*, as well as viruses and fungi, and promotes healing. Nystatin is an antifungal agent and may be used prophylactically or to control a fungal infection. Silver sulfadiazine is incorporated into a number of dressings for antibacterial action, but it is commonly used to prevent wound sepsis and reduce bacterial load in burns. Metronidazole, in gel, cream, or lotion, is effective against bacteria.

65. A: A number of medications can contribute to peripheral edema, especially calcium channel blockers and other antihypertensives (hydralazine, reserpine, beta-blockers, and clonidine) and corticosteroids, as well as hormones (estrogen, testosterone, progesterone), NSAIDs, COX-2 inhibitors, and MAOIs. The patient's medications should be carefully reviewed because some, such as corticosteroids, cause edema and may also impair healing. Drugs that interfere with cell division, such as chemotherapeutic and immunosuppressive agents, and those that inhibit clotting, such as anticoagulants, also can impair healing.

66. C: Prior to debriding a wound covered with dry eschar, the eschar should be softened with autolytic or enzymatic debridement because a moist necrotic wound is easier to debride than a dry one, especially if the eschar is firmly adhered to the wound. Additionally, sharp debridement on wounds covered with dry eschar is contraindicated without a vascular consultation to assess circulation. The eschar should be crosshatched prior to autolytic or enzymatic debridement. A combination of autolytic/enzymatic debridement and sequential sharp debridement is often the most effective.

67. D: Charcot arthropathy may be atrophic or hypertrophic (most common) and can cause joint deformities and fractures. Typical indications include pain and swelling of the foot along with an increase in skin temperature of at least 4°F. Pain may be less severe than expected because of loss of protective sensation. Charcot arthropathy may occur with plantar ulcers or with intact skin and may be misdiagnosed as osteomyelitis. Treatment includes offloading, such as with a total contact cast.

68. B: Silicone polymer gel (supplied in sheets or pads of various sizes and shapes) is placed directly over a maturing scar to treat hypertrophy. Silicone is usually used on small scarring areas or areas where pressure cannot be easily applied. Some people may develop a rash from the silicone, but this usually clears easily if the silicone treatment is withheld for a few days, after which it may be reapplied. Skin breakdown rarely happens unless a rash occurs and the silicone is left in place.

69. D: The Vancouver Scar Scale, which is used to measure scar formation, assesses pigmentation and vascularity as well as pliability and height, with each parameter scored from 0 (normal) to 3–5 (severe), with a higher score indicating a worse scar.

- Pigmentation ranges from normal to hypopigmentation to hyperpigmentation.
- Vascularity ranges from normal to pink, red, and purple.
- Pliability ranges from normal to supple, yielding, firm, banding, and contracture.
- Height ranges from flat to raised > 2mm, raised < 5 mm, and raised > 5 mm.

70. C: The remodeling phase of an acute surgical incision may persist for 1 to 2 years. Usually, the incisional color lightens from red to white over the course of the first year, while the tensile strength gradually increases to about 80% of normal during the same time. During the remodeling phase, it is important for the patient to avoid excessive force or tension on the wound; this may interfere with healing or result in excessive scarring.

71. A: This is a stage I pressure injury. NPIAP stages:

- Stage I: Skin intact with localized non-blanching erythema, decreased skin temperature.
- Stage II: Abrasion, blister, or slightly depressed area with red/pink wound bed but no slough. Partial-thickness superficial skin loss.
- Stage III: Deep full-thickness ulceration that exposes subcutaneous tissue with possible presence of slough; tunneling and undermining but without visibility of underlying muscle, tendon, or bone.
- Stage IV: Deep full-thickness ulceration with extensive damage; necrosis of tissue extending to muscle, bone, tendons, or joints.
- Unstageable: Extent of slough/eschar render ulcer unstageable before debridement.
- Suspected deep tissue injury: Purple/reddish discoloration and boggy, mushy, or firm tissue caused by pressure and/or shear.

72. C: Since bottoming out means that there is less than an inch of support and the patient tends to slide down in bed, which can result in shear, the best choice for this patient is to switch to a dynamic alternating air device, which provides increased support as well as shear and pressure reduction. While this type of surface is more expensive than static devices, it is more moderately priced than low-air-loss or high-air-loss devices.

73. B: Ointments, usually lanolin or petrolatum-based, have the lowest water content and provide the longest duration of moisturizing. They usually must be reapplied once or twice daily. Many oils and lotions are used to increase hydration of the skin. These can include oil baths, which have a minimal effect on hydration but do increase the skin-surface lipids. Lotions have high water content and must be applied 5 to 6 times daily, while creams, which contain water and oil, require application about 4 times daily.

74. A: Atrophie blanche lesions are smooth, white avascular sclerotic skin plaques that occur in about one-third of patients with lower extremity venous disease. They are associated with pain while standing and at rest. The lesions are usually associated with tortuous vessels and hemosiderin staining on the ankles or foot, other indications of venous disease. They may appear similar to scarring from healed ulcers but actually have a high risk for deteriorating into ulcer formation.

75. A: Hammertoes, corns, and claw toes, and small lesions on the toes should be cushioned with tube foam or lambswool. Tube foam can be cut to fit and separates the toes to allow airflow and prevent skin irritation and pressure from the shoe. Diabetic patients should avoid sandals because they leave part of the foot exposed and at risk of trauma. Metatarsal pads relieve pressure on metatarsal heads, and crepe sole shoes provide support for the plantar surface of the foot.

76. B: Sussman Wound Healing Protocol for HVPC for treatment of inflammation requires 60-minute treatments 5 to 7 days per week. The polarity is set at negative, the pulse rate frequency at 30 pps, and the intensity at 100 to 150 V. Edema protocol requires negative polarity, pulse rate frequency of 30 to 50 pps, intensity of ≤ 150 with 60-minute treatments 5 to 7 times per week for 1 week and then 3 times per week for 1 week.

77. D: Ultraviolet C light, which has bacteriocidal properties, can be used to produce a second-degree burn, which causes an inflammatory response that may restart epithelialization in a wound with delayed healing. Other options to promote epithelialization include the use of topical or oral vitamin A and application of electrical stimulation. Topical vitamin A may promote macrophage activity. Some studies have indicated that statins, used to treat high cholesterol, also stimulate epithelialization and have a beneficial effect on healing.

78. D: *Pseudomonas aeruginosa,* characterized by thick, green exudate and foul, musty, fruity odor, is gram-negative aerobic bacilli that favors moist conditions. *P. aeruginosa* is encapsulated, providing protection from antibodies, and produces toxins, enzymes, cytotoxins, and hemolysins that resist phagocytosis and destroy cells of the host. *P. aeruginosa* is an opportunistic infection, invading compromised tissue. It can cause severe infections of virtually all systems and is especially dangerous for those with severe burns or immunosuppression. Additionally, *P. aeruginosa* is resistant to many common antibiotics, and some strains have proven resistant to all antimicrobials.

79. D: Patients experience pain with excessive heating from pulsed short-wave diathermy, which is used to increase blood flow, oxygenation, and metabolic rate, and promote healing. It is also used to relieve pain and edema, so patients should be monitored closely; if pain increases or occurs, the power level should be reduced or air space increased. Care must be taken to avoid any contact with metals or synthetic materials, which increase risk of burns. Electronic devices (watches, hearing aids) should be removed prior to treatment.

80. B: This edema is 2+. Edema is usually checked by pressing the index finger into the tissue on top of each foot, behind the medial malleolus, and over the shin, starting distally and moving proximally to the highest level of edema, comparing both legs. The grading scale is as follows:

- 1+ slight pitting to about 2 mm (persists 10 to 15 seconds).
- 2+ moderate pitting to about 4 mm (persists 10 to 15 seconds).
- 3+ moderate-severe pitting to about 6 mm (persists > 1 minute).
- 4+ severe pitting to 8 mm or more (persists 2 to 5 minutes).

Ostomy Care Practice Questions

1. What percentage of patients with ulcerative colitis will eventually require total colectomy?

a. < 10%
b. 25%
c. 50%
d. 80% to 100%

2. Which of the following is the greatest risk factor for the development of bladder cancer?

a. African American race
b. smoking
c. female gender
d. chronic cystitis

3. When checking aspirant from a J-PEG (jejunostomy) tube, which pH value is consistent with possible gastric migration?

a. 0 to 4
b. > 6.
c. < 6.
d. > 7.5

4. Following surgery for ileal pouch-anal anastomosis (IPAA), which type of anemia must the patient be monitored for?

a. aplastic anemia
b. hemolytic anemia
c. vitamin B12 deficiency anemia
d. folic acid deficiency anemia

5. If a patient is using a wafer skin barrier and stoma bag for management of a low-output enterocutaneous fistula, what is the longest period the appliances should be left in place before changing?

a. 48 hours
b. 3 days
c. 5 days
d. 7 days

6. Which of the following is the appropriate level of responsibility for a 13-year-old child with a colostomy?

a. child is able to empty the pouch independently but not change the appliance
b. child is completely independent in caring for colostomy
c. child requires assistance of school nurse in all colostomy care
d. child is basically independent in caring for colostomy but requires supervision of school nurse

7. The primary difference between a loop transverse colostomy and a double-barrel transverse colostomy is

a. the bowel is continuous in the loop colostomy and divided in the double-barrel.
b. the loop transverse colostomy has a rod and the double-barrel does not.
c. there is essentially no difference.
d. the loop transverse colostomy is usually temporary and the double-barrel is not.

8. Which of the following is the *MOST* likely cause of a patient with Crohn's disease (regional enteritis) complaining of small amounts of diarrhea, increasing Abdominal distension and pain, vomiting, and cramping?

a. abscess
b. fistula
c. colon cancer
d. intestinal obstruction

9. Which over-the-counter medication(s) may increase the risk of pouchitis?

a. antacids
b. acetaminophen
c. NSAIDs
d. loperamide

10. What dietary modification is indicated to manage the acute phase of chronic inflammatory bowel disease (IBD)?

a. low residue, low fat, high protein, and high calorie
b. low residue, low fat, low protein, and high calorie
c. low residue, low fat, and high protein, and low calorie
d. low residue, high fat, and high protein, and high calorie

11. The ideal placement for a stoma for an ileostomy is

a. RUQ.
b. RLQ.
c. LUQ.
d. LLQ.

12. The *MOST* critical indication for total colectomy in a patient with ulcerative colitis is

a. hypocalcemia and anemia.
b. dehydration and electrolyte imbalance.
c. nonresponsive toxic megacolon.
d. erythema nodosum and uveitis.

13. After surgery for Crohn's disease, inflammation

a. never recurs.
b. rarely recurs.
c. recurs in about 10% to 15%.
d. recurs in almost all patients.

14. Infants born with spina bifida should usually begin having intermittent clean catheterization

a. if their diapers are not routinely wet with urine.
b. as newborns.
c. when they are 1 to 2 months old.
d. if they completely stop passing urine.

15. The first goal in management of enterocutaneous fistula is

a. control fluid and electrolyte imbalance.
b. initiate parenteral nutrition.
c. decrease discharge.
d. complete surgical repair.

16. Which foods should be included in the diet of a colostomy patient whose stools are too loose to help thicken the stool?

a. dried fruits, tree nuts
b. broccoli, baked beans
c. applesauce, cheese
d. cabbage, eggs

17. During pregnancy, a woman who has had IPAA should expect

a. no problem with pouch function.
b. increased frequency, urgency, and fecal incontinence.
c. obstruction of the pouch.
d. pouchitis.

18. Following creation of a continent cutaneous fecal diversion with a Koch pouch, how long after surgery is an indwelling reservoir catheter usually left in place?

a. 24 hours
b. 72 hours
c. 5 to 7 days
d. 2 to 3 weeks

19. For how long after surgery should the stoma be routinely measured with each change of appliance?

a. 7 days
b. 1 to 2 weeks
c. 6 to 8 weeks
d. 10 to 12 weeks

20. What postoperative management is indicated if slight mucocutaneous separation is noted on one side of a stoma?

a. fill area with barrier powder and apply a solid wafer skin barrier
b. refer for emergent surgical repair
c. cover area with gauze pressure dressing
d. leave the open area exposed to the air

21. The most common cause of a postoperative enterocutaneous fistula is

a. recurrent disease.
b. anastomotic leak.
c. stomal stricture.
d. functional outflow obstruction.

22. Compared with a two-piece ostomy appliance, a one-piece appliance

a. has a lower profile.
b. is easier to center around the stoma.
c. requires less frequent changing of the skin barrier.
d. requires more manual dexterity.

23. Which of the following is a necessary component of informed consent prior to a procedure?

a. names of assisting staff members
b. beginning and ending times
c. risks and benefits of procedure
d. facility statistics regarding procedure

24. After creation of a Hartmann's pouch, the patient should be advised to expect

a. rectal bleeding.
b. rectal discharge of mucoid material.
c. rectal discharge of fecal material.
d. no rectal bleeding or discharge.

25. Which type of stoma involves bringing both the proximal and distal ends of the bowel to the skin surface at different places on the abdomen?

a. loop
b. split
c. double-barrel
d. trephine

26. How far away from the skin surface should the external fixation device of a percutaneous endoscopic gastrostomy (PEG) tube be placed to prevent buried bumper syndrome?

a. 1 to 2 cm
b. 2 to 3 cm
c. 4 to 5 cm
d. flush with the skin

27. Which is the surgical procedure of choice for a patient with ulcerative colitis?

a. ileal pouch-anal anastomosis (IPAA)
b. ileostomy
c. sigmoid colostomy
d. transverse loop colostomy

28. Which of the following actions is correct in working with a 44-year-old Asian female patient who states a surgical preference but plans to leave the decision to family members?

a. recognize that cultural values regarding individualism vary and respect the patient's right to be guided by family
b. try to convince the patient to assert herself
c. tell the family that the patient should be the one to make the decision
d. ask the ethics committee to intervene

29. What is the *BEST* solution for an ileostomy patient who develops peristomal irritation from adhesive because of the frequent need to change appliances?

a. leave area exposed for an hour after removing appliance
b. rinse the skin with water only
c. use a medical adhesive remover to cleanse the skin prior to cleaning with water
d. change to a different brand of appliance

30. Considering the PLISSIT (Permission, Limited Information, Specific Suggestions, and Intensive Therapy) model for communicating about sexuality, what is the *BEST* response if a patient tells a nurse that he does not want to talk about sexual issues?

a. "If you change your mind, I can give you some information that may be helpful."
b. "You don't need to feel embarrassed."
c. "That's fine. We won't discuss it further."
d. "You really should reconsider."

31. The initial intervention for a slightly prolapsed stoma is

a. manual reduction.
b. apply cold compress.
c. laparoscopic local repair.
d. resiting of the stoma.

32. A 15-year-old ostomate who wants to participate in team sports should be advised to

a. avoid all team sports.
b. wear a stoma cup during sporting activities.
c. wear a plastic stoma shield during sporting activities.
d. wear a support garment during sporting activities.

33. Which stage of Elisabeth Kübler-Ross's stages of grief is a patient likely experiencing if she doubts the legitimacy of her doctor's recommendation and says she wants to see a different doctor regarding the need for a colostomy?

a. anger
b. denial
c. depression
d. bargaining

34. Which type of pouch is able to hold the greatest volume of fecal material?

a. N pouch
b. J pouch
c. W pouch
d. S pouch

35. The food enzyme alpha-D-galactosidase (Beano) is effective to prevent gas from

a. complex sugars.
b. lactose.
c. fiber.
d. wheat products.

36. What is the MOST important factor in helping the patient work toward rehabilitation?

a. realistic goals
b. patient-identified goals
c. nurse-directed goals
d. patient confidence

37. Which of the following is the *BEST* method to prevent depression in ostomates?

a. provide thorough information about ostomy care
b. provide emotional support
c. refer patient to support group
d. enlist the help of family and friends

38. By what age does a patient with familial adenomatous polyposis usually begin to develop cancer?

a. 10
b. 20
c. 30
d. 40

39. Which symptoms are *MOST* consistent with Hirschsprung disease, which is diagnosed during childhood?

a. episodes of vomiting
b. diarrhea
c. chronic constipation
d. foul stools with ribbon-like appearance

40. The *BEST* response to a patient who is concerned that she only has a bowel movement every 3 days after surgery for colorectal cancer with a formation of a descending colostomy is

a. "You probably need to take a stool softener."
b. "You should begin to do daily irrigations."
c. "Most people only have stools every 3 days with a colostomy."
d. "Unless the stool is very hard, then every 3 days is probably normal for you."

41. When siting a stoma, the stoma on an obese patient is usually

a. higher than usual.
b. lower than usual.
c. the same as for nonobese patients.
d. more medial than for other patients.

42. When arranging for a visit for a patient from another ostomate, which criterion or criteria are *MOST* important to match?

a. ethnicity
b. age and gender
c. age and social background
d. educational background

43. Preoperative screening for a patient with inflammatory bowel disease that caused severe diarrhea and bleeding should include which of the following?

a. cardiac enzyme tests
b. liver function tests
c. renal function and electrolytes tests
d. lung function tests

44. How often should a PEG tube be flushed during continuous feedings to prevent blockage?

a. every 4 to 6 hours
b. every 6 to 8 hours
c. every 1 to 2 hours
d. every 2 to 4 hours.

45. Prior to surgery, information about the surgery and stoma care is *BEST* provided

a. upon patient request.
b. routinely in written and oral form.
c. by giving patients lists of Internet resources.
d. by video format.

46. When irrigating a colostomy, what is the optimal time for instillation of fluids?

a. 15 to 20 minutes
b. 10 to 15 minutes
c. 1 to 5 minutes
d. 5 to 10 minutes

47. How much normal saline should be used to irrigate a blocked ureteral stent after urostomy surgery?

a. 1 to 2 mL
b. 5 to 10 mL
c. 10 to 20 mL
d. 30 to 60 mL

48. The best time to change a urostomy appliance is

a. at bedtime.
b. 1 hour after eating.
c. after breakfast in the morning.
d. in the morning before eating or drinking.

49. The most frequent postoperative complication for patients undergoing colorectal surgery is

a. bleeding.
b. stomal ischemia.
c. hypovolemia and hypotension.
d. nausea and vomiting.

50. Following surgery for a continent ileostomy, how long should the patient expect to have a catheter in place for continuous drainage?

a. 24 to 48 hours
b. 2 to 3 days
c. 3 to 4 weeks
d. 1 to 2 months

51. A patient who has undergone an IPAA with formation of a J pouch should usually expect to pass stool

a. 1 to 2 times daily.
b. 3 to 4 times daily.
c. 6 to 8 times daily.
d. 10 to 12 times daily.

52. Which test is indicated to confirm a functional outflow obstruction after IPAA?

a. endoanal ultrasound
b. defecating pouchogram
c. MRI
d. CT scan

53. A patient with colorectal cancer characterized by tenesmus is likely to have which type?

a. right-sided cancers
b. left-sided cancers
c. rectal cancers
d. anal cancers

54. When considering patient characteristics related to readiness to learn, which of the following factors should be assessed first?

a. physical factors
b. experience
c. mental/emotional status
d. knowledge/education base

55. Which type of ostomy is *LEAST* likely to require routine irrigation?

a. sigmoid colostomy
b. ileostomy
c. transverse colostomy
d. descending colostomy

56. Which of the following teaching tools is most effective for patients with low literacy skills?

a. posters
b. videos
c. materials written at fourth-grade level
d. slide show presentations

57. How much drainage would be anticipated within 24 hours with a small/medium output fistula?

a. < 100 mL
b. < 150 mL.
c. 150 to 500 mL
d. > 500 mL

58. If excessive leakage occurs around a PEG tube, which is the *BEST* intervention?

a. change PEG tube, inserting a larger size
b. change to a J-PEG tube
c. change the PEG tube, inserting a smaller size
d. apply skin barrier and try to identify cause

59. When inserting a balloon replacement gastrostomy tube, what position should the nurse place the patient in?

a. flat supine
b. head of bed, elevated 30 degrees
c. head of bed, elevated 45 degrees
d. head of bed, elevated 60 degrees

60. When emptying a closed-system drain, the drain device (such as Hemovac) should be held

a. even with the shoulder.
b. above the level of the wound.
c. even with the level of the wound.
d. below the level of the wound.

61. After formation of an orthotopic neobladder, what is the longest period of time, day or night, that a patient should go without emptying the bladder?

a. 3 hours
b. 4 hours
c. 5 hours
d. 6 hours

62. The *MOST* likely cause of concentrated foul-smelling urine and decreased urinary output from a urostomy is

a. urinary tract infection
b. dehydration.
c. pouchitis.
d. ureteral blockage.

63. What is the *MOST* likely cause when a patient with a urostomy develops a pruritic macular rash with red borders and moist red and yellow centers in the peristomal area after wearing an appliance for a week?

a. bacterial infection
b. allergic dermatitis
c. fungal infection
d. herpes

64. What is the *PRIMARY* purpose of using an introducer tip for clean intermittent catheterizations?

a. reduce urethral trauma
b. reduce discomfort associated with catheterization
c. facilitate catheterization
d. reduce incidence of urinary tract infections

65. In the postoperative period after formation of an orthotopic neobladder, how often should the Foley catheter be routinely irrigated?

a. every 8 hours
b. every 2 hours
c. every 4 hours
d. every 12 hours

66. Which of the following is a contraindication for an orthotopic neobladder?

a. older than 65 years
b. tumor spread to proximal prostatic urethra
c. hypertension
d. stress incontinence

67. Chronic pouchitis with IPAA is classified as episodes of pouchitis lasting

a. > 2 months.
b. > 4 months.
c. > 2 weeks.
d. > 4 weeks.

68. When draining a continent cutaneous fecal diversion, about how far should the catheter be inserted into the stoma?

a. 1 inch
b. 2 inches
c. 5 inches
d. 10 inches

69. A BMI of 17 in a 25-year-old woman with inflammatory bowel disease probably indicates that the patient is

a. underweight.
b. of normal weight.
c. overweight.
d. obese.

70. Prior to ileostomy takedown, the patient should probably expect what type of prep?

a. irrigations
b. clear fluids for 24 hours and NPO for 6 to 12 hours
c. laxatives
d. laxatives and irrigation

71. The most common extraintestinal manifestation associated with ulcerative colitis is

a. anemia.
b. uveitis.
c. erythema nodosum.
d. rheumatologic disorders, such as arthritis.

72. The most common site for desmoid tumors associated with familial adenomatous polyposis is

a. trunk.
b. abdominal wall
c. intra-abdominal/mesentery.
d. extremity.

73. Which of the following therapies may be *MOST* helpful in improving anal sphincter control to relieve incontinence?

a. biofeedback
b. acupuncture
c. relaxation exercises
d. hypnosis

74. Surgical intervention is indicated for interstitial cystitis

a. upon initial diagnosis.
b. when other treatments have failed.
c. when pain persists for more than 2 years.
d. upon patient request.

75. A dietary obstruction in a patient with an IPAA is usually resolved by

a. increasing fiber in the diet.
b. fluids only for 24 hours.
c. irrigation.
d. stimulant suppository.

76. Patch testing to determine if an ostomate is allergic to a product is done by placing a small amount of the product

a. on the forearm for 24 hours.
b. on the inner thigh for 24 hours.
c. on the face for 48 hours.
d. on the abdomen for 48 hours.

77. Following abdominoperineal resection of the rectum, what is the usual cause of severe dyspareunia in a female patient?

a. inadequate lubrication
b. anxiety
c. scar tissue
d. nerve damage

78. What is the initial step in managing a blocked PEG tube?

a. check for kinks in the tubing
b. squeeze and roll the tubing to dislodge blockage
c. aspirate fluid
d. instill 5 to 10 mL of warm water

79. Following creation of an orthotopic neobladder, patients should be closely monitored for

a. metabolic alkalosis.
b. metabolic acidosis.
c. respiratory alkalosis.
d. respiratory acidosis.

80. Which of the following is considered a contraindication for continent cutaneous urinary diversion?

a. kidney disease
b. spina bifida
c. paraplegia
d. hypothyroidism

Ostomy Care Answers and Explanations

1. B: About 25% of patient with ulcerative colitis will eventually require total colectomy. Ulcerative colitis manifests with superficial inflammation of mucosa of colon and rectum, causing ulcerations in the areas where inflammation has destroyed cells. These ulcerations, ranging from pinpoint to extensive, may bleed and produce purulent material. The mucosa of the bowel becomes swollen, erythematous, and granular. Onset is usually between 15 and 30 years of age, and there is a genetic component. Ulcerative colitis may affect only the rectum (ulcerative proctitis), the entire colon (pancolitis), or only the left colon (limited or distal colitis).

2. B: Smoking: Greatest risk factor; smokers have twice the rate of bladder cancer as nonsmokers. Carcinogens in lungs enter bloodstream, are filtered by kidneys, and concentrated in urine, damaging bladder lining. **Race/Genetics:** Caucasian rate is twice that of others. Family clusters occur. **Age/Gender:** More than 70% are older than 65 years. Men's rate is twice that of women. **Chronic cystitis:** Especially with indwelling catheters or bladders left intact after urinary diversion. **Other:** Exposure to aniline dye and aromatic amines and other organic chemicals, previous bladder cancer, congenital defects, chemotherapy/radiation, arsenic in drinking water, parasites, and low fluid consumption.

3. A: The pH of gastric fluids is usually 0 to 4, so this finding may indicate proximal migration of the J-tube. The pH in the small intestine is usually less than 6 while a higher pH such as greater than 7.5 may indicate pulmonary migration. A marked increase in intestinal residual volume may indicate migration. If that occurs, then feedings should be held for at least an hour before pH testing is done. Gastric aspirant is usually curdled and clear to white, while intestinal aspirant may be brownish/greenish because of bile staining.

4. C: Patients who have undergone IPAA must be monitored for both iron deficiency anemia and vitamin B12 deficiency anemia. Because part of the ileum is used to form the pouch, patients may not absorb adequate vitamin B12. Iron deficiency anemia may occur with pouchitis or inflammation of the rectal cuff. Patients should have annual evaluation that includes complete blood cell count, folate, ferritin, and vitamin B12 levels, and liver function tests. Patients should be advised of dietary sources of iron and vitamin B12 and of symptoms of deficiency.

5. D: While the appliances for a low-output enterocutaneous fistula may appear intact because of the relatively small amount of drainage, the appliances should be removed at least every 7 days so that the skin about the fistula can be examined. Generally, appliances are changed every 2 to 3 days. The skin should be washed gently with warm water, avoiding soap because it may cause drying and irritation of the skin. The skin should be thoroughly air dried (a hair dryer on low heat or air may be used) before a new appliance is applied.

6. B: By about the sixth grade (age 11 or 12), the child should be completely independent in caring for a colostomy. In early adolescence, children strive to be in control and should be allowed autonomy whenever possible. Children should be independent in emptying the pouch by kindergarten. By age 6, children should be independent in care at school, but ostomy supplies should be at school and the school nurse knowledgeable about ostomy care. Children should be given increasing levels of responsibility each year.

7. A: The primary difference between a loop transverse colostomy and a double-barrel transverse colostomy is that the bowel is continuous in a loop colostomy and divided in a double-barrel colostomy. The loop colostomy sometimes has a rod or bridge placed, but this is not always done. In both cases, because part of the colon as well as the rectum and anus are retained, the colostomies may be done as temporary procedures with reanastomosis done at a later time.

8. D: These symptoms are indicative of intestinal obstruction, which may be partial or complete. Obstructions are common because strictures develop in the bowel from repeated ulcerations of mucoid tissue. Chronic diarrhea is common, and some diarrhea may persist even with obstruction, depending on the location and degree of obstruction. Other common complications include abscesses, fistulae (especially from the small bowel to the skin), fissures, and malnutrition. Lesions associated with Crohn's disease are most common in the distal ileum and ascending colon.

9. C: NSAIDs are associated with increased risk of pouchitis and discontinuing them may relieve symptoms. If pouchitis persists, the initial treatment of choice is ciprofloxacin 400 mg twice daily for 2 weeks. If nonresponsive, then the ciprofloxacin may be combined with metronidazole 400 mg twice daily for 4 weeks. Pouchitis is characterized by increased frequency and urgency of stools and sometimes bleeding. Most patients have only 1 episode of pouchitis, but it may become chronic and relapsing in some patients.

10. A: During the acute phase of chronic inflammatory bowel disease, patients should be advised to stay on a low-residue, high-protein, low-fat, and high-calorie diet. This type of diet is digested primarily in the jejunum, allowing the bowel to rest. Patients should especially avoid foods that cause irritation, as this may be quite individual, and should be sure to drink at least 8 glasses a day because patients often become dehydrated. In severe case of IBD, patients may require parenteral nutrition.

11. B: The ideal placement for a stoma for an ileostomy is in the right lower quadrant, about 2 inches below the waist, although this may vary if there are folds or scar tissue that precludes this placement. The stoma should be conveniently placed, avoiding bony prominences, so that the patient can easily see the stoma and manage care independently, and so that an appliance can be easily applied. The site should be marked prior to surgery, usually by the surgeon or enterostomal therapist, and discussed with the patient.

12. C: With toxic megacolon, inflammation extends through the mucous lining of the intestines into the smooth muscle of the muscularis, which controls peristalsis. Because the intestinal ability to contract becomes impaired, the colon distends. Symptoms include weakness, fatigue, fever, pain, vomiting, and distention. Treatment includes insertion of a nasogastric tube for decompression, IV fluids, electrolyte replacement, corticosteroids, and antibiotics, but if the condition does not respond within 1 to 3 days, then total colectomy is usually performed.

13. D: After surgery for regional enteritis, the inflammation almost always returns at some point. Within 5 years, almost 30% of patients have experienced recurrence, so medical management remains very important to try to control symptoms and control progression of the disease. About 50% of patients with regional enteritis eventually need surgery of some type. One common procedure to relieve strictures in the small intestine is laparoscopic strictureplasty, which opens narrowed portions of the intestines. In some cases, a segment of the small bowel is removed, but others require ileostomy.

14. B: Most children with spina bifida have normal function of the kidney and ureters, but the kidneys may become damaged because of urinary retention and abnormalities associated with the lower urinary tract; therefore, clean intermittent catheterization (CIC) should begin after birth because, if bladder function is normal, urination is reflexive in the infant, but the child may have sphincter impairment or other abnormalities, so catheterization can help to determine whether the child has residual urine. The infant should have urodynamic studies done as soon as possible to determine whether CIC should be continued.

15. A: The initial goal of enterocutaneous fistula management is to control fluid and electrolyte imbalance. Dehydration is frequent with high-output fistulae, and patients may develop hyponatremia and hypokalemia with metabolic acidosis. Parenteral nutrition, if necessary, should be initiated after the fluid/electrolyte balance is re-established. Up to 90% of patients with enterocutaneous fistulae develop malnutrition, and if patients are unable to obtain adequate nutrition orally, then enteral or parenteral feedings may be indicated, depending on the site of the fistula.

16. C: Patients with colostomies must learn to balance the diet to help control stool consistency. If stools are too loose, the patient should include foods that may be constipating.

Foods that promote constipation/thickening of stools include:

- Fruits*:* applesauce, bananas.
- Proteins*:* cheese, creamy peanut butter.
- Starches*:* potatoes (without skins), rice, pasta, whole wheat bread, tapioca pudding, marshmallows.

Foods that cause diarrhea/loosening of stools include:

- Fruits: juices (especially apple and prune juice), prunes, fresh fruit.
- Vegetables: broccoli, cabbage, raw vegetables.
- Other: spicy foods, fried foods, baked beans, sugar-free gum.

17. B: During pregnancy, a woman who has had IPAA often experiences increased frequency of stool, urgency, and fecal incontinence, especially during the night. Women should be advised to use a skin barrier about the anal area at night if incontinence occurs to help prevent skin irritation. Problems tend to increase throughout the pregnancy and are most pronounced during the third trimester when pressure increases on the small bowel. Normal functioning generally returns after delivery.

18. D: Following creation of a continent cutaneous fecal diversion with a Koch pouch, an indwelling reservoir catheter is usually left in place for 2 to 3 weeks to decompress the pouch in order to give the sutures time to heal. Fecal output from the indwelling catheter must be carefully measured as patients often lose large amounts of fluid postoperatively, sometimes up to 2000 mL daily in addition to fluids lost through urine and perspiration. Fluid intake must be adequate to prevent fluid and electrolyte imbalance.

19. C: The stoma is initially swollen, moist, and shiny after surgery and may be oval or circular in shape, but the size and shape of the stoma will change as healing occurs and swelling recedes, so the stoma should be measured with each appliance change for the first 6 to 8 weeks after surgery until the size and shape stabilizes. Usually cut-to-fit appliances are used after surgery, but standard sizes can generally be used once the stoma has reached its final size.

20. A: Mucocutaneous separation may occur if there is too much tension on the intestine or if the tissue was not adequately approximated. If the mucocutaneous separation is slight, then it does not generally require surgical repair. When applying an appliance, the open separated area should be filled with barrier powder or alginate and then covered with a solid wafer skin barrier to protect it from fecal drainage. It should be monitored closely to ensure that it is healing and further separation is not occurring.

21. B: The most common cause of postoperative fistula is anastomotic leak, which results in infection and/or abscess. About 50% of fistulae originate from an abscess, so careful observation for signs of infection is important as early antibiotic treatment (often metronidazole) and drainage of the abscess may prevent development of fistulae. Patients may exhibit fever, cramping, abdominal pain, localized swelling, and erythema before the fistula opens to the surface and begins to drain purulent and then fecal material.

22. A: A one-piece appliance (skin barrier wafer and drainage pouch together) has a lower profile, so this may be the choice of a patient who is concerned about appearances. Also, the one-piece appliance requires less manual dexterity because the bag does not need to be snapped into place and there is less chance of leakage. However, it is more difficult to center the one-piece appliance over the stoma, and the entire appliance with the skin barrier must be removed in order to change the bag.

23. C: Patients/family should be apprised of all reasonable risks and any complications that might be life-threatening or increase morbidity, as well as benefits. The American Medical Association has established guidelines for informed consent:

- Explanation of diagnosis.
- Nature of, and reason for, treatment or procedure.
- Risks and benefits.
- Alternative options (regardless of cost or insurance coverage).
- Risks and benefits of alternative options.
- Risks and benefits of not having a treatment or procedure.
- Providing informed consent is a requirement of all states.

24. B: To create a Hartmann's pouch, the intestine is severed, usually with removal of a part of the distal segment because of a cancerous lesion. The proximal end is brought through the abdominal wall to form a stoma for fecal drainage. The nonfunctioning distal end of the colon with the rectum intact is stapled or stitched to close and then left in place, forming a nonfunctioning pouch, but rectal mucoid discharge still occurs periodically. Fecal discharge only occurs if the colon was inadequately cleansed prior to surgery.

25. B: The split or divided stomas (Devine procedure) are formed by bringing both the proximal and distal ends of the bowel to the skin surface at different places on the abdomen. The ileostomy is formed from the proximal portion (ileum) and a nonfunctioning colostomy with the distal portion (colon). This is usually a temporary procedure after a subtotal colectomy to allow healing, and reanastomosis is done at a later time.

26. A: The external fixation device of a PEG tube should be placed 1 to 2 cm above the skin surface to prevent excessive tension that may result in buried bumper syndrome (BBS), in which the internal fixation device becomes lodged in the mucosal lining of the gastric wall, resulting in ulceration. Rotating the PEG tube also helps to prevent BBS. Typical symptoms of BBS include increasing abdominal pain and difficulty infusing the feeding solution. If BBS occurs, the PEG must be replaced.

27. A: The surgical procedure of choice for a patient with ulcerative colitis is ileal pouch-anal anastomosis (IPAA) (restorative proctocolectomy), although patients with fulminant ulcerative colitis requiring emergency surgery usually receive an ileostomy and may then receive the procedure at a later date. The IPAA procedure retains the anal sphincter, creating a reservoir to contain stool. There are a number of different approaches to IPAA, but newer laparoscopic, minimally invasive procedures reduce recovery time.

28. A: Under the American Nurses Association Code of Ethics, autonomy and self-determination are viewed within the broad context of diverse cultures. The idea of individualism is less important in some cultures, so the nurse must respect and appreciate the patient's right to be guided by her family. Trying to convince the patient to assert herself may just lead to emotional conflict. This is not an appropriate concern for the ethics committee because the woman is not being forced to comply with family decisions but chooses to do so.

29. C: The adhesive backing on ostomy appliances can be irritating to the peristomal skin, especially if adhesive residue remains after removing the appliance, so the best solution is to gently cleanse the skin of residue with a medical adhesive remover. Then the skin can be cleansed with water or a mild soap and water, but most soaps should be avoided as they may result in drying and further irritation of the skin. Virtually all appliances have some type of adhesive backing, and leaving the skin exposed is not practical for an ileostomy, which may drain continuously.

30. A: The best response is, "If you change your mind, I can give you some information that may be helpful." This leaves the opening for the patient to reconsider and provides a reason, without assuming that the patient is "embarrassed." It is also not coercive. PLISSIT model:

A. Level one: Permission for the patient to have feelings or attitudes and to do or not do something.
B. Level two: Limited Information is given.
C. Level three: Specific Suggestions are made.
D. Level four: Intensive Therapy is given.

31. B: A slightly prolapsed stoma may respond to a cold compress applied to the stoma. If this is not successful, then a manual reduction may be successful. The prolapsed bowel must be carefully monitored for color and signs of obstruction because it may become edematous, impairing circulation, and may incarcerate. Care must be taken when applying an appliance to choose one that decreases mechanical irritation. If the prolapse is more severe, then surgical intervention may be indicated.

32. C: Ostomates should be able to participate in sports activities once their stomas are well healed, but those involved in sports that may involve body contact should use a plastic stoma shield over the appliance (and under clothing) for extra protection. The protective shield is usually secured with a belt. Support garments are intended for those with parastomal hernias but may also provide some protection during sporting activities. Stoma cups contain absorbent material and are often worn while patients are bathing but provide little protection.

33. D: The patient is experiencing the stage of bargaining, during which patient/family may change doctors, trying to change the outcome. People grieve individually and may not go through all stages, but most go through at least 2 stages. Kübler-Ross's 5 stages of grief include:

- Denial: disbelieving, confused, stunned, detached, repeating questions.
- Anger: directed inward (self-blame) or outward.
- Bargaining: If–then thinking. (If I go to church, then I will heal.) Trying to find a different outcome.

- Depression: Sad, withdrawn, tearful, crying, but beginning to accept loss.
- Acceptance: Resolution and acceptance.

34. C: The W pouch is able to hold the largest volume of fecal material, although it may not be appropriate for a patient with a small pelvis. The S pouch is rarely used now, replaced by the W and J pouch, because of problems with spontaneous evacuation, and it is the most difficult pouch to construct. There is no pouch titled the N pouch. In general, all pouches function in similar manners, and the type of pouch a patient is given often relates to surgeon preference.

35. A: The food enzyme alpha-D-galactosidase (Beano) prevents gas related only to complex sugars but not sorbitol, lactose, fiber, or wheat. Antiflatulent agents both disperse gas and prevent formation of gas bubbles. Simethicone (Mylanta, Phazyme) allows small gas bubbles to gather into larger ones, making them easier to expel by belching. Certain activities may increase swallowing of air and development of gas, including smoking, using drinking straws, chewing gum, and talking while eating.

36. B: Patient-identified goals are the most important factor in helping a patient work toward rehabilitation. The nurse should explore with the patient what he/she wants to be able to resume or wants to change because this can serve as the basis for a plan of action. The nurse should make a point of linking training and education to reaching the goals the patient has identified and helping patients to use their skills and knowledge to do the same.

37. A: While all of these are important, studies have indicated that the greatest cause for depression is lack of adequate education and preparation for self-care. Patients want to know how long recovery should take, how to maneuver changes in roles during different recovery phases, what treatments will be prescribed, what complications might occur, and how to handle complications. Patient education should be individualized so that the amount of information and the method of delivery are appropriate for the patient.

38. B: Familial adenomatous polyposis (FAP) is an inherited autosomal-dominant syndrome in which people develop hundreds to thousands of colorectal polyps between ages 5 and 40 years, with cancer usually in 1 or multiple polyps by about age 20. Between 20 and 40, virtually every FAP patient develops cancer. A genetic factor predisposes people with this genetic mutation to other malignancies, especially in duodenum and stomach. Identifying FAP before colorectal cancer develops is critical as prophylactic colectomy may be indicated with high risk.

39. D: Hirschsprung disease is a congenital disorder in which infants are born without intestinal ganglion nerve cells in part or the entire colon, causing mechanical obstruction. It may be an acute life-threatening or chronic condition. Symptoms associated with childhood diagnosis include:

- Foul stools with ribbon-like appearance.
- Thin, poorly nourished appearance and anemia.
- Chronic cycles of constipation with palpable fecal masses in abdomen.
- Abdominal distension with visible peristaltic waves.

Hirschsprung disease accounts for about 25% of all neonatal obstructions, is 4 times more common in males than females, may have a genetic link, and is more common in children with Down syndrome.

40. D: While stools from an ascending colostomy are quite liquid, those from a descending colostomy are more normal in consistency. People who had regular bowel movements before surgery may be well controlled after surgery, but the frequency of bowel movements varies widely from a 2 to 3 times a day to every 1 to 3 days. Some people need to irrigate or even take stool softeners while others do not. Patients should try to establish a routine. Some people find that certain foods or drinks or even digital stimulation promotes emptying of the bowel.

41. A: The stoma of an obese patient is usually placed higher than usual in the abdomen because the girth of the abdomen and abdominal folds associated with obesity make placement in the usual position difficult. Additionally, the stoma must be positioned so the patient is able to see it to carry out routine care, and this often requires higher placement as well. The stoma should be placed in the rectus abdominis muscle below the waistband. The patient should be assessed in different positions for siting.

42. B: The most important criteria when matching a patient with another ostomate are age and gender. While male and female patients have similar concerns, there are some differences, and patients may feel more embarrassed or intimidated about expressing their concerns to a patient of the opposite gender. People at different ages also face different challenges. If patients have self-identified as part of the LGBT community, matching for sexual orientation as well as age and gender may help patients feel more comfortable.

43. C: The severe diarrhea resulting from inflammatory bowel disease may result in dehydration and electrolyte imbalances that can adversely affect renal function, so these tests should be done preoperatively. Other routine blood tests include the complete blood cell count and coagulation studies. ECG may be indicated for those at risk for heart disease or with a history of heart disease. Routine chest x-rays are usually not indicated but may be ordered for patients older than 60 years or those undergoing major colorectal surgery.

44. A: During continuous feedings, the PEG tube should be flushed with 30 mL of warm water every 4 to 6 hours, whenever feedings are stopped for a period of time, and before and after any administration of medications. Medications should never be added to the feedings. Administer medications separately with a flush of about 10 mL of water between them. Pills should be crushed completely and dissolved if possible. Liquid preparations of medications should be used when available.

45. B: While it is important to respond to a patient's request for information, education about surgery and stoma care should be routinely provided to all patients in both oral and written form. Patients are often quite anxious and may not remember everything that is discussed, so they should be provided written materials to review. Internet resources, such as the United Ostomy Associations of America, can also provide valuable information, and videos are especially useful to demonstrate procedures.

46. D: When irrigating a colostomy, the optimal time for instillation of fluids is about 5 to 10 minutes. A slower rate is not necessary, but instilling fluids too fast may cause cramping and leaking around the cone tip, so the flow should be adjusted with the manual control. The bottom of the bag should be level with the patient's shoulder, and once the fluid has been instilled, the cone should be held in place for about 15 seconds and then removed slowly. The amount of fluid used varies (250 to 1500 mL), but is usually around 500 mL.

47. B: A ureteral stent is a piece of thin, pliable tubing that is inserted inside of the ureter to maintain patency during the postsurgical period when edema of the ureter could cause occlusion. These tubes protrude through the stoma and are often different lengths or color-coded to differentiate which ureter they serve, and each should be drained and monitored separately. A blocked stent may be irrigated with 5 to 10 mL of normal saline, using care not to apply tension or pressure that may dislodge the tube.

48. D: Changing the pouch: If possible, change the pouch in the morning before eating or drinking when urine flow is decreased, or wait 2 hours after eating or drinking. Remove pouch. Stand or sit as comfortable, keeping a paper towel or gauze to absorb drops of urine. Cleanse peristomal tissue, dry skin, and apply new bag, using mirror to guide if necessary.

The two main types of urostomy pouches are the one-piece with attached skin barrier and the two-piece with a skin barrier and pouch that detaches. The pouches have drains at the bottom for emptying and to attach a nighttime drainage tube.

49. D: Because of the manipulation of the intestines during colorectal surgery, the most common postoperative complication is nausea and vomiting, sometimes related to paralytic ileus, so patients should be carefully monitored for bowel sounds. Patients may return from surgery with a nasogastric (NG) tube for decompression, and this should be monitored for patency. Patients who develop paralytic ileus may require insertion of the NG tube if one is not in place. Additionally, antiemetics may help relieve symptoms.

50. C: Continent ileostomy:

First 3 to 4 weeks: Prevent excessive pressure that could cause perforation or tearing by using constant drainage. If catheter plugs or falls out, replace immediately. The catheter needs to be irrigated with 1 ounce of tap water several times daily, letting liquid drain back out. Next phase: Continuous draining stops and intermittent draining begins, usually every 2 hours during the day with constant drainage at night. Gradually the time interval between draining increases and constant night drainage stops, but the pouch may need to be drained once or twice during the night.

51. C: While there is individual variation, most patients should expect to pass stool 6 to 8 times daily. The capacity of a J pouch is about 400 mL, but stool is usually loose or quite soft. About half of patients with IPAA need to evacuate at least once during the night. Weakness of the sphincter may result in fecal leakage or incontinence. The patient should be advised to cleanse and dry the anal area frequently. If leakage occurs, a skin barrier, such as zinc oxide, may be indicated to prevent maceration.

52. B: With functional outflow obstruction, which may be caused by abnormalities in pelvic descent during passing of stool or compression during filling of the pouch, endoscopy is usually normal, so a defecating pouchogram is indicated to confirm the diagnosis. Symptoms include decreased frequency of defecation and persistent difficulty defecating. Some patients may have good results from biofeedback, but others may need to catheterize the pouch with a medina catheter. If the condition is not resolved, then some patients may have pouch revision.

53. C: Rectal cancers are characterized by rectal bleeding, tenesmus (feeling as though defecations are inadequate or incomplete), and a change in bowel habits. Bleeding is usually bright red, but patients with hemorrhoids may assume the bleeding is related to the hemorrhoids. Patients often exhibit weight loss, but this occurs with advanced disease, sometimes because patients reduce intake because of persistent problems with defecation. Mucus discharge is also common. Pain is a late and uncommon symptom and may occur with obstruction.

54. D: Knowledge/education: The nurse should begin by assessing patients' knowledge about their disease, condition, or treatment, and their cognitive ability. Physical factors: Manual dexterity may be required to complete a task, hearing or vision deficits may impact ability, and complex tasks may be too difficult for some because of weakness or cognitive impairment. Experience: Experience with learning can vary widely and is affected by their ability to cope with changes, their personal goals, motivation to learn, and cultural background. Mental/emotional status: Anxiety, fear, or depression about the condition can make learning very difficult because people cannot focus on learning.

55. B: The stool from an ileostomy is quite liquid as is stool in an ascending colostomy. The stool from a transverse colostomy is usually soft and mushy and generally passes without the stimulation of irrigation. Irrigations are used to stimulate or control passage of stool primarily from descending or sigmoid colostomies because the remaining colon absorbs more liquid than other types of colostomies, and the stool is firmer. In some cases, drinking coffee or juice or using a mild laxative may also stimulate passage of stool.

56. B: Videos are more effective than written materials for those with low literacy or poor English skills. Focused viewing in which the nurse discusses the purpose of the video presentation prior to viewing and then is available for discussion after viewing can be very effective. Patients and/or families are often nervous about learning patient care and are unsure of their abilities. Allowing the patients/families to watch a video demonstration or explanation first and allowing them to stop or review the video presentation can help them to grasp the fundamentals before they have to apply them.

57. C: Volume (drainage) classification for fistulas:

- Low-output fistulas: Drains less than 150 mL in 24 hours.
- Small to medium output: Drains 150-500 mL in 24 hours.
- High output: Drains more than 500 mL in 24 hours.

Different classifications systems are used with fistulas, which are also classified as simple or complex. Anorectal fistulas are often classified according to the Parks classification system. Anorectal (or cryptoglandular) fistulas are the most common type of fistulas, occurring most frequently in female patients.

58. D: If excessive leakage occurs around a PEG tube, the best intervention is to apply skin barrier to protect the skin from maceration and try to identify the cause. Some drainage is normal in the first few days after placement, but a large amount of leakage usually indicates a complication, so just changing the type of tube or the size of tube will not solve the problem. Complications could include infection, hypergranulation, and buried bumper syndrome. A J-PEG should be inserted if the drainage results from feeding intolerance.

59. B: Insertion of balloon replacement gastrostomy tube:

1. Gather supplies, position patient to 30°.
2. Inject 20 mL of sterile water into balloon port to check leaks; withdraw water and retain filled syringe.
3. Move external disk to near distal end and catheter tip.
4. Cleanse peristomal area with NS in spiral movement. Dry skin.
5. Insert tube gently to premeasured distance and inflate balloon.
6. Gently pull tube until resistance met. Slide external bumper to 1.5 cm from skin surface.
7. Rotate tube in circular motion to ensure free rotation.
8. Use 30-60 mL syringe to aspirate gastric content. Flush tube with water.
9. Apply barriers and mark exit measurement.

60. D: Closed drainage systems use low-pressure suction to provide continuous gravity drainage of wounds. Drains are attached to collapsible suction reservoirs that provide negative pressure.

Management includes daily dressing changes around tube insertion site, inspection of skin for inflammation or drainage, monitoring type and amount of drainage from drain, and emptying device by holding it lower than the wound, opening the plug, draining, squeezing all air out to reestablish suction and negative pressure, and reinserting plug. There are two closed drainage systems that are in frequent use: Jackson-Pratt and Hemovac.

61. D: A patient with a neobladder should not go longer than 6 hours without emptying the neobladder because the capacity usually does not exceed 500 mL and may be smaller in some patients, especially in the weeks after surgery. Leakage is common, especially in the first year after surgery as the bladder expands, and some patients may continue to have leakage, so emptying the bladder on a regular schedule may help to control leakage. Patients must do pelvic floor exercises to strengthen sphincter control.

62. A: Concentrated foul-smelling urine and decreased urinary output are consistent with urinary infection. In some cases, the urine may be cloudy with purulent material evident, or hematuria may occur. Patients may complain of back pain, fever, and chills, especially if the infection spreads to the kidneys.

Urinary tract infections are often a recurrent problem for patients with urostomies, so patients should be advised to monitor urine characteristics and drink at least 2 L of fluid daily.

63. C: A macular rash with red borders and moist red and yellow centers is consistent with a fungal infection. This is a common occurrence if moist conditions exist under an appliance, which can occur with leakage of urine under urostomy appliances if left in place too long. Appliances should be changed about every 3 days so the skin can be examined. Nystatin powder is usually used to treat peristomal fungal infections.

64. D: The distal portion of the urethra is often contaminated with fecal bacteria, such as *E. coli*, so the introducer tip is inserted into the urethra to provide a barrier to this area of the urethra, and then the catheter is fed through the introducer tip and into the bladder. The introducer tip is often used in closed systems but is increasingly recommended for clean intermittent catheterization in order to reduce urinary tract infections.

65. C: After formation of the neobladder, the bowel segment used for creation of the neobladder continues to a produce a significant amount of mucus, which may obstruct the Foley catheter, increasing tension on suture lines. Thus, irrigating the Foley on a routine basis every 4 hours is essential. Some patients may require additional irrigations as well. If mucus is allowed to collect in the neobladder for longer periods, irrigation is more difficult and time-consuming, as it should be continued until the irrigant returns clear of mucus.

66. D: Stress incontinence is a contraindication for orthotopic neobladder because the patient lacks adequate sphincter control. Tests for sphincter muscle control should be completed as part of the workup to determine whether a patient is a candidate for the neobladder. Other contraindications include tumor spread to distal prostatic urethra or bladder neck (female), renal or liver function impairment, Crohn's disease, cognitive impairment, and inadequate mobility and/or manual dexterity.

67. D: Acute pouchitis, characterized by increasing frequency of stools, urgency, cramping, and incontinence, lasts less than 4 weeks, and chronic lasts more than 4 weeks. Rectal bleeding and fever are rare but can occur, and the degree and extent of symptoms do not always correlate with the extent of inflammation. Some patients may develop relapsing pouchitis, classified as 3 or more relapses within a year or relapse within a month of completing antibiotic therapy. In some cases, patients may become antibiotic dependent or refractory.

68. C: To drain a continent cutaneous fecal diversion, the catheter should be inserted about 5 inches into the stoma. Initially, the pouch needs to be drained about every 3 hours, but this time period extends as the pouch heals and stretches. Most patients are able to drain the pouch only 3 to 4 times daily and are able to go through the night without draining unless they have eaten a late meal that stimulates peristalsis.

69. A: Body mass index (BMI) scores for adults 20 years and older:

Below 18.5	Underweight
18.5 - 24.9	Normal weight
25.0 - 29.9	Overweight
30 and above	Obese

BMI is a measurement that uses height and weight as an indicator of obesity/malnutrition. This cannot be used alone to diagnose obesity as body types differ considerably. Women often have more body fat than men. Tables are available to make calculations simple, but the BMI can be calculated manually.

BMI formula: Weight (lb)/ [Height (in)]^2 x 703

Metric BMI formula: Weight (kg) / [Height (m)]^2.

70. B: While preps may vary according to physician preference, in general, ileostomy takedown requires much less preparation than colostomy takedown, so the most common preparation is clear liquids for 24 hours and then the usual NPO the night before surgery. Colostomy takedown, on the other hand, requires complete cleansing with laxative agents and may require the patient to sit in the bathroom for a number of hours until any discharge is clear of all fecal material.

71. D: The most common extraintestinal manifestation associated with ulcerative colitis is rheumatologic disorders, such as arthritis, arthralgia, and ankylosing spondylitis. Osteoporosis may also occur, especially for those treated with corticosteroids. Anemia affects almost 1 in 5 patients both because of bleeding from the gastrointestinal tract and iron and/or vitamin B12 deficiency. Other manifestations can include primary sclerosing cholangitis and various ocular disorders, such as uveitis, iritis, and episcleritis. Skin problems are also common and can include pyoderma gangrenosum, psoriasis, and erythema nodosum.

72. C: About 70% of desmoid tumors, which are encapsulated fibromatous tumors that are locally invasive, occur in the intra-abdominal area/mesentery of those with FAP. The tumors are not metastasizing and many do not progress, so they can be monitored but often require no treatment. However, those in the small intestine may result in blockage and are a leading cause of death in those with FAP. Surgery appears to stimulate development of desmoid tumors, so they may arise after surgery.

73. A: Biofeedback has been useful for improving both urethral and anal sphincter control, with about 66% of patients who use feedback, demonstrating improvement. Techniques vary widely, and biofeedback is often used along with Kegel exercises and other therapies. For anal sphincter control, a common method is to insert an anal or vaginal probe and then ask the patient to contract the pelvic floor muscles. The patient receives computer-generated feedback, usually through some type of graph, and tries to improve performance.

74. B: Surgery is usually the last intervention for interstitial cystitis, used after all other treatments have failed and scar tissue has rendered the bladder size inadequate. Treatments may include oral medications (ibuprofen, tricyclic antidepressant, and pentosan). Other treatments include nerve stimulation, bladder distention, and bladder instillations. Surgery that leaves part of the bladder intact, such as bladder augmentation and fulguration, often results in recurrence of symptoms. Cystectomy with ileal conduit formation is a last resort option.

75. B: dietary obstruction in a patient with an IPAA is usually resolved by ingesting only fluids for 24 hours. Massaging the abdomen and walking about may also help to dislodge the obstruction. Obstruction usually results from too much fiber in the diet, such as from eating raw fruits and vegetables. Patients with IPAA should avoid high fiber foods and should eat cooked fruits and vegetables. If the obstruction does not resolve within 24 hours, the patient should seek medical assistance.

76. D: Patients often have to try different types of products in order to find those that are most effective, so they should use a patch test before changing, especially if they tend to have many sensitivities. For the patch test, a small amount of product is applied to a site on the abdomen distant from the stoma. If it is not self-adhering, it should held in place with hypoallergenic tape. After 48 hours, the product should be removed and the skin examined for signs of irritation.

77. C: Dyspareunia may occur in both males and females, but is much more common in females and is almost always the result of scar tissue. Patients often experience pain at the vaginal meatus and at the far end of the vagina, so insertion and thrusting of the penis during sexual intercourse may be very painful. Some patients may also experience vaginismus, making intercourse almost impossible. Patients experiencing dyspareunia should seek medical advice.

78. A: Opening an occluded PEG tube involves first checking for kinks or obvious problems, such as a patient rolling over onto a tube. Next, the nurse should try milking the tube and then attaching a 30-60 mL syringe and aspirating fluid. After that, 5-10 mL of water can be slowly instilled (over about a minute) and aspirated a number of times to try to loosen occlusion. After clamping for 10-15 minutes, the flushing procedure can be repeated with warm water. If the water fails, a multienzyme cocktail or pancreatic enzyme and sodium bicarbonate solution may succeed.

79. B: Following creation of a neobladder, patients are at increased risk of developing hyperchloremia metabolic acidosis because the segment of bowel used to create the bladder absorbs sodium chloride to balance the hypo-osmolar urine coupled with increased serum hydrogen. Patients may be advised to increase dietary sodium intake, although some patients may need sodium bicarbonate for 2 or 3 months. Blood gas analysis should be done frequently. A chronic state of hyperchloremic acidosis may result in osteoporosis.

80. A: Kidney disease is a contraindication for a continent cutaneous urinary diversion because the ileum, which is used to create the pouch, retains some absorptive abilities, so some waste products that should be excreted in the urine are reabsorbed back into the circulatory system and return to the kidneys for filtering. However, if kidney disease is present, the kidneys often cannot adequately filter the increased waste products. If kidney function is inadequate, then the diversion of choice is the urostomy.

Share Your Story!

It's Your Moment, Let's Celebrate It!

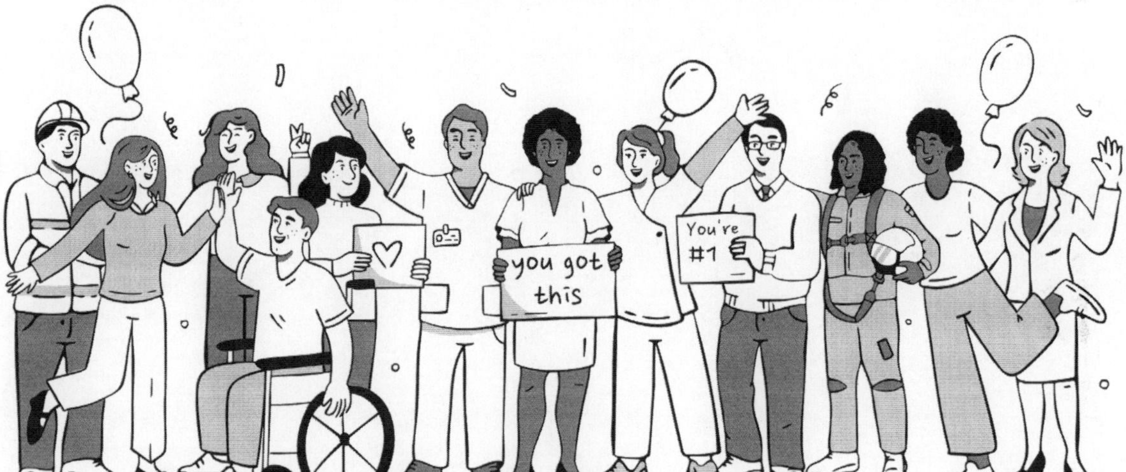

Share your story @mometrixtestpreparation